Practical Guide to Mental Health Nursing

Practical Guide to Mental Health Nursing

W Vimala Samson
MSc (Nursing) RN, RM, MBA (EdM)
Reader, Mental Health Nursing
Dr G Sakunthala College of Nursing
Thiruvanai Kovil, Trichy-5
Tamil Nadu, India

Forewords
V Kanagaraj
G Gopalakrishnan
BG Kulkarini

JAYPEE BROTHERS MEDICAL PUBLISHERS (P) LTD
New Delhi • London

Jaypee Brothers Medical Publishers (P) Ltd.

Headquarters

EMCA House
23/23-B, Ansari Road, Daryaganj
New Delhi 110 002, India
Landline: +91-11-23272143,
+91-11-23272703+91-11-23282021,
+91-11-23245672
E-mail: jaypee@jaypeebrothers.com

Corporate Office
Jaypee Brothers Medical Publishers (P) Ltd.
4838/24, Ansari Road, Daryaganj
New Delhi 110 002, India
Phone: +91-11-43574357
Fax: +91-11-43574314
E-mail: jaypee@jaypeebrothers.com

Overseas Off ce
JP Medical Ltd.
83, Victoria Street, London
SW1H 0HW (UK)
Phone: +44-20 3170 8910
E-mail: info@jpmedpub.com

EU GPSR Authorised Representative
Logos Europe, 9 rue Nicolas Poussin
17000, La Rochelle, France
Phone: +33 (0) 6 67 93 73 78
E-mail: Contact@logoseurope.eu

Website: www.jaypeebrothers.com
Website: www.jaypeedigital.com

Inquiries for bulk sales may be solicited at: jaypee@jaypeebrothers.com

Practical Guide to Mental Health Nursing

First Edition: 2011

Reprint: **2025**

ISBN 978-93-5025-158-4

Printed in India

Dedicated to

Mr Samson Selvaraj
and
my son
S Nisi Williams

Foreword

The author deserves to be congratulated for preparing the *Practical Guide to Mental Health Nursing*. I feel an immense pleasure in presenting the Foreword for the Practical Guide brought out by W Vimala Samson.

Psychiatric nurses use a number of interpersonal and communication skills to help clients cope up with their psychiatric problems. Psychiatric nurses have a unique role to play in their professional career. They promote psychological health on aspects of "holistic approach" to the individual, family and community. The knowledge related to mental health nursing is essential to guide the students to move towards the wellness of patient's health.

The author has taken genuine interest to bring out this Practical Guide, which would be useful as an "informative material" to the students as well as to the teachers to enhance their knowledge, aptitudes and practices in their professional career.

The Practical Guide is prepared on the basis of Indian Nursing Council's revised syllabi for BSc and MSc nursing students. It is designed for developing an understanding of the modern approach to mental health problems with special emphasis on therapeutic intervention for individual, family and community. I believe that it would help open up for the reader an exciting world of important goal.

V Kanagaraj MD, DCH, DLO
Secretary and Managing Director
of Dr G Sakunthala College of Nursing
Trichy, Tamil Nadu, India

Foreword

The *Practical Guide to Mental Health Nursing* has been brought out with an increase in awareness regarding the various roles a psychiatric nurse can play. A guide to clinical practice, provides answers of how to's for mental health professionals and nursing students enabling them to frame clinical question in a way that supports and to be used as mental health nursing practical guide. To equip her for this commendable task, an urgent need was felt in molding the curriculum at various levels of nursing.

This Practical Guide authored by *W Vimala Samson* is a concrete step toward this end. It contains authentic information to a whole range of psychiatric assessment and various roles of mental health nurse in providing a holistic care for the psychiatric disorders. The role of a psychiatric nurse in applying nursing care plan, treatment modalities in administration of psychotherapeutic drugs and various therapies have been dealt with extensively and efficiently to meet the curriculum requirements of diploma, graduate and postgraduate nursing courses.

The Practical Guide is an excellent resource that fosters and promotes mental health nursing practical knowledge at all levels of nursing students in facing their practical examinations and also enable them to equip themselves better for their future endeavors.

G Gopalakrishnan MD (Psych)
Professor of Psychiatry and CEO
Sowmanasya Hospital and
Institute of Psychiatry
Trichy, Tamil Nadu, India

Foreword

It is my proud privilege to foreword this *Practical Guide to Mental Health Nursing*. Mental health is one of the major components of total health. In present-day stressful life, all of us have to balance, maintain and promote our mental health. Mental health services are facing much more challenges. Social stigma related to mental health still prevails. We, mental health professionals, especially psychiatric nurses, should take bold step to make awareness among people to broaden their knowledge and utilize the available mental health services to keep themselves mentally healthy.

Mental health challenges are increasing at rapid pace. We nurses have to update our theoretical as well as clinical knowledge to cope up with present day demands and to get definitely mastery over clinical care. We need to have dedication, devotion and self understanding. Mental health nursing has a global demand especially Indian psychiatric nurses. As we develop humanitarian care, our aim is to provide quality academic services to our students and make them graduate bedside nurses.

It is not an easy task to write a book especially covering practical aspects. The author has taken a lot of pain to write this book by keeping in mind the requirements of Indian Nursing Council syllabi. This book contributes everything in meeting clients mental health needs and helps deliver safe and appropriate mental health services at institution and community. The author has taken keen interest not to miss any point related to practical aspects in clinical areas.

The Practical Guide will help students, teachers and professionals to overcome clients mental health problems and withstand for present need in providing quality care to all clients suffering from various behavioral disorders. Author has tried by adding supportive, innovative, creative and critical thoughts in form of *Practical Guide to Mental Health Nursing* to provide a comprehensive care to individual, family and community.

I congratulate the author in taking a lot of effort to publish this book. I strongly recommend all nursing libraries and professional's shelves and students need to reserve a copy of this book.

BG Kulkarini MSc (Nursing)
Professor of Psychiatry
Bengaluru, Karnataka, India

Preface

The *Practical Guide to Mental Health Nursing* forms one part of a comprehensive system developed by the author to facilitate the practical knowledge of mental health nursing. It is designed for diploma, BSc and MSc nursing students as well as mental health professionals.

The Practical Guide is heavily illustrated to enrich an awareness regarding the various roles a psychiatric nurses can play to perform and to provide curative, preventive, promotive and rehabilitative care to all patients with psychiatric disorders in the hospitals.

It has been especially prepared to meet the curriculum requirement formulated by the Indian Nursing Council, a new revised syllabus for mental health nursing practical examination. This is an effort to bridge the gap between theory and practice for mental health professionals.

The Practical Guide consists of nine chapters, which deal with the followings:

1. Format for assessment of history collection, mental status examination, general and physical examination, neurological assessment, and process recording for patient with psychiatric disorders.
2. Role of a nurse in administration of drugs to patients with psychiatric disorders.
3. Application of psychiatric nursing process on patient with mental illness to provide holistic care.
4. Theories of physical, social, cognitive, psychosexual, emotional, and moral development.
5. Case record for psychosis, neurosis, mental retardation and epilepsy.
6. Case work on child guidance clinic, community psychiatry, and National Mental Health Programme.
7. Role of a mental health nurse, preparation for and assisting with treatment modalities and various therapies used in mental disorders.
8. Counseling patient and family.
9. Field trip and observational visit on outpatient department, mental retarded rehabilitation, psychiatric rehabilitation and de-addiction centers.

This book will prove to be extremely useful for Diploma, BSc nursing, and MSc nursing students in facing their practical examination and also enable them to equip themselves better for their future endeavors. A list of references has been furnished at the end of the guide for further reading.

All constructive suggestions from the readers in making this Practical Guide more valuable and helpful will be earnestly solicited.

W Vimala Samson

Acknowledgments

I praise the Almighty for His grace and abundant blessing He has showered upon me. His immiscible presence and guidance had helped me to complete this *Practical Guide to Mental Health Nursing*.

I expressed my sincere thanks to Dr V Jayapal MS, FICS, President, Dr V Kanagaraj MD, DCH, DLO, Secretary and Managing Director of Dr G Sakunthala College of Nursing for their ceaseless guidance, thoughtful comments, constant encouragement and for being a driving force for the successful completion of this Practical Guide.

My sincere thanks to Dr G Gopalakrishnan MD (Psych), Professor of Psychiatry and CEO, Sowmanasya Hospital and Institute of Psychiatry, Trichy-2, for his timely support and constructive suggestions.

My sincere gratitude to Prof Mrs BG Kulkarini Madam, for her expert guidance and support with valuable suggestion.

I expressed my sincere thanks to my Principal Mrs Shantham Sweet Rose, MSc, PhD, for her support and for her valuable suggestions.

I owe my sincere gratitude to my mentor, enlighting personality Professor Mrs Irene Light, MSc(N), PhD, for her expert guidance, encouragement, and motivation to complete this practical guide.

My sincere heartfelt thanks to Mrs CS Sowndaram, MA, MPhil, PhD in Psychology and Mrs R Punithavathi, MSc(N), for her guidance and support.

I also take the opportunity to express my sincere appreciation to my husband Mr Samson Selvaraj, my son S Nisi Williams, my mother Mrs A Maryrajakantham, my sister Mrs W Shyamala Selvakumar, and Mrs W Nirmala Monfort.

I am deeply moved to thank the family members Mr C Arokiadoss, Mrs A Sagayamary, Mrs A Sarala Omprakash and Mrs Jaculine Cyrilraj, and to my friends who are always a source of inspiration and strength whose immense prayers and blessings helped me to carry out this Practical Guide in a successful manner.

I also express my deep sense of gratitude to M/s Jaypee Brothers Medical Publishers (P) Ltd, New Delhi for having readily consented to publish this book on Mental Health Nursing.

Contents

Chapter 1

ASSESSMENT FORMAT

MENTAL HEALTH NURSING

OVERALL OBJECTIVE

The student is able to provide curative, preventive, promotive and rehabilitative care to patients with psychiatric disorders in the hospitals. It will help students to develop advanced skills for nursing intervention in various psychiatric conditions.

SPECIFIC OBJECTIVE

The student is able to:

1. Describe the current trends and scope in mental health nursing.
2. Describe the national mental health nursing act, programme and mental health policy.
3. Demonstrate therapeutic communication skills in all interactions.
4. Explain the principles and standards of mental health nursing.
5. Provide comprehensive care to patients with psychiatric disorders.
6. Explain dynamics of human behaviour in different situations.
7. Describe the magnitude of psychiatric problems and trends in psychiatric care.
8. Explain assessment, etiology, psychopathology, clinical manifestations, evaluation and management of various psychiatric disorders of child, adolescence and old age.
9. Apply different principles and concepts into every aspect of nursing care.
10. Explain treatment modalities, various therapies, guidance and counseling used in mental disorders and role of the nurse.
11. Provide holistic care to individual with various psychiatric disorders in the hospital using nursing and other techniques.
12. Develop desirable attitudes.

HISTORY TAKING OF PATIENTS WITH MENTAL ILLNESS

A. SOCIODEMOGRAPHIC DATA

1. Name:
2. Father's/Spouse's name:
3. Address: Rural/Urban
4. Age:
5. Sex:
6. Language — Mother tongue:
   Other Languages:
7. Marital status: 1. Single 2. Married 3. Separated
   4. Divorced 5. Widow 6. Widower
   7. Other
8. Education:
9. Occupation:
10. Income (per month):
11. Religion:
12. Informant: Relationship with the patient:

B. PRESENTING COMPLAINTS

Includes onset of present illness, duration of present illness, course, precipitating factors, Aggravating, maintaining, and/or relieving factors, if any:

1. ________________________________
2. ________________________________
3. ________________________________
4. ________________________________
5. ________________________________
6. ________________________________

C. HISTORY OF PRESENT ILLNESS

Duration of total illness: (wks/months/yrs)

Current: episode/exacerbation

Mode of onset: Abrupt < 48 hr/Acute < 1 wk/Sub acute 1- 2 wk/Insidious

Course: Continuous/Episodic/Unclear/Fluctuating/Deteriorating/Improving.

Precipitating factors: (describe)

Description:

(In cases of long duration, divide into initial, middle and recent phases)

(Chronological account, describe major abnormal behaviour, associated problems like homicide/suicide/disruptive behaviour, thought contents as expressed in speech/ writing, major mood states, abnormal perceptions and experiences, biological functioning, interpersonal and social functioning, occupational functioning, changes in daily life, etc.)

(Scheme for substance abuse/dependence cases)

Mode of initiation, early pattern of intake, progression, salience, tolerance, craving, physical withdrawal features, pattern of use in recent past, medical complications (including accidents, neuro psychiatric problems, interpersonal problems, socio-economic problems (including debts, if any), occupational problems , problems with law, earlier attempts to abstain, reason for consultation, motivation for abstinence, etc. (In case of multi substance use, describe separately for each substance)

Treatment History:

- (Magi co-religious/other systems
- (Homeopathy/Ayurveda/Allopathic (Medical))
- Psychiatric (Present)

Pharmacotherapy:

List drugs as far as possible from to dose response side effect.

ECTS:

- Psychotherapy:
- Family interventions:
- Rehabilitative measures:

Negative History:

- Major features that are usually present in the given syndrome
- Other associated major syndromes
- Other major Psychiatric illness Organic causes
- Substance uses.

D. PAST HISTORY (CHRONOLOGICAL ACCOUNT SINCE CHILDHOOD)

Describe each episode briefly, with onset, major features, course and duration, interventions level of recovery).

- Psychiatric illness:
- Medical illness:

E. FAMILY HISTORY

1. Family tree (pedigree) (Draw the tree for 3 generations on both sides in cases of genetic importance.
2. Describe each family member briefly (Relationship, age, education, occupation, age at death, mode of death, health status physical and psychological, major personality traits, relationship with client, include other significant members).
3. Details of family functioning
   a. Type of Family: (Nuclear/Joint/Other)
   b. Social economic status: (Upper/Middle/Lower)
   c. Leadership
   d. Communication
   e. Child rearing practices
   f. Interpersonal relationships
   g. Social position
   h. Social support systems
   i. Other.

History of illness in family: Psychiatric: Similar illness, Other illness, Other major behavioral problems like delinquency, personality problems, suicide, substance use, epilepsy, mental retardation.
Medical: (especially hereditary).

F. PERSONAL HISTORY

Birth and development:

- Antenatal period: Uneventful/Eventful (specify)
- Birth History: (Full term/premature/post mature/normal/forceps/cesarean/delayed birth cry/any other problems.
- Postnatal history: Uneventful/eventful (specify)
- Physical health during infancy: Good/poor (specify)
- Immunization schedule: completed/not completed
- Developmental milestones: Normal/delayed
- Childhood health: Normal/abnormal/trauma/fever/convulsions/any other illness
- Behavioral and emotional problems: Nail biting, enuresis, sleep walking, temper tantrums, Stammering)
- Emotional problems in adolescence: Running away/delinquency/Smoking/drug taking/overweight/identity problems.
- Home atmosphere during adolescence: Satisfactory/unsatisfactory
- Parental lack: Yes/No (Dead, separated for more than one year, habitually absent from home

- Anomalous family situation: Yes/No (Step parent adoption status)
  Comments:

G. EDUCATIONAL HISTORY

Age of beginning: Age of finishing:
Grade reached:

(if discontinued, reason for it)
Relationship with teachers:
Relationship with school mater (include nickname, bully/butt of jokes):
Position in class: (Top, Middle, Low)
Special abilities:
Active participation in games: Yes/No
Other extra curricular activities:

H. OCCUPATIONAL HISTORY

Work record: Satisfactory/unsatisfactory frequent changes of jobs: Yes/No
Work position: Rising/Failing/Stationary
Age at the time of starting to work:
Jobs held in the past (in chronological order, with wages, dates, reasons for change).
1. ____________________
2. ____________________
3. ____________________
4. ____________________
5. ____________________

Present Job: Duration:

Satisfied with work: Yes/No (Reasons for dissatisfaction)

I. SEXUAL HISTORY

Information about sex (How acquired, of what kind, how received, adequacy of knowledge, attitude towards, opposite sex)
Masturbation: Age of starting: Frequency (Guilt if, any)
Sexual experiences: (Home/Hetero/Pre and extramarital/Preference)
Any complaints including *Dhat*:

J. MENSTRUAL HISTORY

Age at menarche/how regarded/regularity/duration/cycle/amount/physical/ emotional problems

LMP:

Menopause: (Age/climacteric symptoms)

K. MARITAL HISTORY (GENOGRAM/FAMILY OF PROCREATION)

Date/Year of marriage: Arranged/Affair

Spouse: Age, Education, Occupation, Personality

Marital relationship: Satisfactory/Unsatisfactory

Contraceptive practices:

Children: Chronological list of children/miscarriage and still births (age, education, occupation, personality for each child, relationship with client).

L. PREMORBID PERSONALITY

Give details and cite examples from patients past life.

i. Social relations
ii. Intellectual activities: Hobbies and interests:
iii. Mood (Cheerful, strung on, optimistic, pessimistic, stable, fluctuating, etc.)
iv. Character
   a. Attitude to work and responsibility
   b. Interpersonal relationships
   c. Standards in moral, religious, Social and health matters.
   d. Energy and initiative
v. Fantasy life: (Day dreaming - content and frequency)
   Habits:
   Eating foods/patterns:
   Sleeping patterns:
   Excretory functions:
   Alcohol consumption:
   Tobacco consumption:
   Self-medication with drugs:

MENTAL STATUS EXAMINATION OF PATIENTS WITH MENTAL ILLNESS

1. General Appearance and Behavior

Appearance: Looking one's age/order/younger

Level of growing: Normal/shabbily dressed/over dressed

Level of cleanliness: A adequate/inadequate/overtly clean

Level of consciousness: Fully conscious and alert/drowsy/stuporous/comatose

Mode of entry: Came willingly/Persuaded/Brought physically

Cooperativeness: Normal/More than so/Less than so

Eye-to-Eye contact: Maintained/Difficult/Not maintained

Psychomotor activity: Normal/Increased/Decreased

Empathy: Easy/Difficult/Sustained/Unclear

Rapport: Spontaneous/Difficult/Not established

Quality of rapport: Good/Poor

Gesturing: Normal/Exaggerated/Bizarre

Posturing: Normal posture/Catatonic posture

Other movements: Mannerisms/Stereotypic/Tremors/EPS/AIMS/Preservation

Other catatonic phenomena: Automatic obedience/Negativism/Cooperation/Waxy flexibility/Echoproxia.

Details:

2. Speech

Initiation: Spontaneous/speaks when spoken to/minimal/mute

Reaction time: Normal/Delayed/Shortened/Difficult to assess.

Speed: Normal/Slow/Rapid/Not clear

Output: Normal/Increased/Decreased/Variable

Pressure of speech: Present/Absent

Volume: Normal/Increased/Decreased

Tone: Normal variation/Monotonous

Manner: Normal/Highly formal/In appropriately familiar

Relevance: Fully relevant/Sometimes off target/Irrelevant

Coherence: Fully coherent/Over elaborate, digressive, circumstantial speech/Some Loosening of associations/Incoherent

Others: Rhyming/Punning/Echolalia/Preservation/Neologism

Sample of speech (in response to open ended questions)

3. Thought

Tempo: Normal/Racy thoughts/Flight of ideas/Retarded thinking/Muddled/Unclear thinking/Thought block/Circumstantiality's/Tangentially.

Form: Adequate/Wooly and vague thinking/Loosening of associations/Gross Formal thought disorder (FTD) (Refer to sample of speech for examples of disorders of tempo and form)

4. Obsessive-compulsive Phenomena

(Major content/Interference/Distress/Recognition of in appropriateness/Resistance)

Obsession: (Thought/Doubt/Impulse/Image/Rumination)

Compulsion: (Yielding/Controlling/Mental compulsion)

Examples: Thought alienation phenomena (Thought insertion/withdrawal/Thought broadcast).

Thought contents: (Idea/over valued idea/delusion)

(Worthlessness/Helplessness/Hopelessness/Guilt/Ill health)

Poverty/Nihilistic/Hypochondriac/Death wish/Suicidal Grandiose Ability and Identity/Reference/Ideas/Control/Influence/Persecution/Bodily change/Religious/Bizarre)

(Single/Multiple/Simple/Elaborate/Systematized/Nonsystematized/Mood congruent/Incongruent/Degree of distress/Interference with work/Reaction to phenomena)

Examples:

5. Mood

Subjective:

Objective:

(Predominant mood state/Other major moods/Range/Reactivity/Quality (Mood/Communicability/Liability/Appropriateness/Congruence/Emotional expression):

Normal/Blunted flattened/Made affect)

Description:

6. Perception

Hallucination: Pseudohallucination		Single/multiple
Auditory: Illusion		One modify/Many modalities
Visual depersonalizations		Elementary/Partially formed/Fully formed
Olfactory:		
Gustatory	Derealization	Occasional/Continues
	Deja Vu phenomena	Mood congruent/Mood incongruent
Tactile		Degree of distress
Somatic		Reaction to phenomena special

7. Cognitive function

Attention: Normally aroused/Aroused with difficulty

Digit forward: Digit backward:

Concentration: Normally sustained/Sustained with difficulty/Distractible

100 - 7

40 - 3

20 - 1

Name of months (backwards)

Name of week days (backwards)

8. Orientation

Time : Approximate time/Day-night/Date/Day/Month/Year/........

Place : Kind of place/Area/City...........

Person : Self/Close associate/Hospital staff

9. Memory

Immediate (Same test as for attention)

Recent: Recent happenings (last meal/visitors, etc.)

Verbal recall	after 5 min	after 10 min
3 unrelated objects/	....	....
5 unrelated objects/	....	....
Imaginary address if 5 times	....	....
Visual recall 3 or 5 unrelated Objects	....	....
Remote:		
Personal events	....	....
Impersonal events	....	....
Illness related events	....	....

10. Intelligence

Comprehension: Simple commands/Complex commands

Vocabulary: Common objects/Uncommon objects/Parts of objects

General fund of information: ....

Arithmetic ability: Mental arithmetic, Written sums ....

Details:
Abstraction: Normal/Concrete/Personalized/Bizarre
Interpretation of proverbs
Similarities between paired objects:
Dissimilarities between paired objects:

11. Judgment

Intact/Impaired.
Personal: (Sense of personal capability/worth and planning of future)
Social test: (Sense of what is socially and culturally acceptable)
(Prediction of one's own behavior in imaginary situations)

12. Insight

Awareness of abnormal behavior/experience	Yes/May be/No
Attribution to physical causes	Yes/May be/No
Recognition of personal responsibility	Yes/May be/No
Willingness to take treatment	Yes/May be/No

Grade (1 = No insight, 6 = Full insight)
Any other information: (Motivation/Willingness for treatment:
Diagnosis:

GENERAL AND PHYSICAL EXAMINATION

Name, Age and Sex
Ward Unit: Income:
Date: Time:

GENERAL EXAMINATION

BODY TYPE: Asthenic/Athletic

Dysthymic, Pyknic:
Temperature:

Anemia: Pale, Conjunctiva Tongue Pallor of Nail Beds

Nourishment: Good, Moderate, Poor, Emaciated, Dehydrated.

Jaundice: Sclera, Palate, Skin

Hair: Distribution Normal, Scanty, Hirsutism Alopecia Healthy, Unhealthy.

Cyanosis:

Clubbing:

Skin: Dry, scaly, glistening patches, others

Lymph nodes:

Breast:

Other details:

Edema:

Thyroid:

General nervous system:

Level of consciousness:

Handedness:

Speech:

Posture:

Cranial nerves:

Fundi		**Pupils**	
L	**R**	**L**	**R**

Others

Motor system:

Power:

Tone:

Nourishment

Co-ordination:

Cerebellar system:

Involuntary movements:

Gait:

Sensory system:

Reflexes Superficial: Deep tendon: Infantile:

Skull

Spine

Cardiovascular System:

Pulse Carotids Radial Dorsalis Pedis

JVP

BP

Cardia:

Respiratory System

Abdomen

Contour Mass:

Tenderness Organs

Rigidity Fluid:

Genitourinary and Rectal Examination:

Bones and Joints:

Other Observation:

Behavioral Observation:

Mute:	Restless
Stuporose	Aggressive
Psychomotor Retardation	Overtalkative
Suicidal Risk	Escaping Tendencies:

Identification Marks

1.

2.

Date: Signature of the Examination Doctor

Name:

NEUROLOGICAL ASSESSMENT

DEFINITION

Neurological examination is a method of obtaining specific data in relation to the function of a patient's nervous system.

INDICATION

Neurological observations are required to monitor and evaluate changes in the nervous system by indicating trends, thus aiding diagnosis and treatment which in turn may affect prognosis and rehabilitation .

HISTORY

Questioning relatives, friends or the ambulance team is an essential part of the assessment of the unconscious or the unco-operative patient.

Has the patient sustained a head injury leading to admission, or in the preceding weeks?

- Did the patient collapse suddenly?
- Did limb twitching occur?
- Have symptoms occurred in the preceding weeks?
- Has the patient suffered a previous illness?
- Does the patient take medication?

NEUROLOGICAL OBSERVATIONS AND ASSESSMENT

The following describes a full neurological assessment:

Special consideration:

- A fully conscious patient will respond to questions quickly and is alert to events occurring around him. As his condition deteriorates he may display irritability, lack of concentration and uncooperative behavior.
- A comatose state is one in which the patient fails to respond to verbal and painful stimuli, fever and pain commonly cause confusion, disorientation and irritability.
- To prevent the patient from falling, stand by the side of the patient during the test.
- The patient's cultural and educational background influences his ability to answer test questions.

EQUIPMENT

1. Cotton applicator	Assesses patients response to light touch.
2. Needle	Assesses patient's response to pain
3. Test tube containing hot and cold water	Assesses temperature sensation.
4. Reflex hammer	
5. Vials containing coffee or vanilla extract, sugar salt.	Assesses olfactory nerve
6. Tongue blade	
7. Penlight	
8. Snellen chart	
9. Tuning fork	
10. Thermometer	
11. BP apparatus	
12. Stethoscope	

NERVOUS SYSTEM—HISTORY
1. HEADACHE

- Onset-sudden/gradual.
- Frequency
- Severity
- Character—aching/throbbing
- Associated features—vomiting/visual disturbance
- Site
- Relieving factors—analgesics
- Precipitating factors—stooping/coughing
- Timing, e.g. morning

2. VISUAL DISORDER

Onset
Frequency
Duration
Precipitating factors

Impairment:	One/both eyes	
	Total/partial visual loss	
	Whole/partial field loss	
Diplopia:	gaze direction where maximal	
Hallucinations:	field involved –	formed, e.g. images (real)
		Unformed, e.g. shapes or zig-zags.

3. LOSS OF CONCIOUSNESS

- Onset
- Frequency

Duration precipitating factors

- Tongue biting
- Incontinence
- Limb twitching
- Alcohol/drug abuse
- Head injury
- Cardiovascular or respiratory symptoms

4. SPEECH DISORDER

- Onset
- Frequency
- Duration
- Difficulty in articulation
- Difficulty in expression
- Difficulty in understanding

5. MOTOR DISORDER

- Onset
- Frequency
- Duration
- Precipitating factors, e.g. walking
- Relieving factors, e.g. rest

- Incoordination-balance
- Weakness-progression/clumsiness/difficulty in walking/leg stiffness
- Involuntary movement.

6. SENSORY DISORDER

- Onset
- Frequency
- Duration
- Precipitating factors, e.g. walking, neck movement
- Relieving factors, e.g. rest
- Pain
- Numbness/Tingling
- Site.

7. SPHINCTER DISORDER

- Onset
- Frequency
- Duration
- Bladder and anal
- Difficulty in control—incontinence/retention.

8. LOWER CRANIAL NERVE DISORDER

- Onset
- Frequency
- Duration
- Precipitating factors, e.g. neck movement, head position
- Deafness/Tinnitus—uni/bilateral.
- Vertigo—rotation of surrounding
- Balance/Staggering—direction
- Swallowing difficulty
- Voice change.

9. MENTAL DISORDER

- Onset
- Frequency
- Duration
- Memory/Intelligence—deterioration

- Personality/Behavior—change.
- Nervous system—examination

Neurological disease may produce systemic signs and systemic disease may affect the nervous system. A complete general examination must, therefore, accompany that of the central nervous system. In particular, note the following:

- Temperature
- Blood pressure
- Neck stiffness
- Pluse irregularity
- Carotid bruit
- Cardiac murmurs
- Cyanosis/respiratory insufficiency
- Evidence of weight loss
- Breast lumps
- Lymphadenopathy
- Hepatic and splenic enlargement
- Prostatic irregularity
- Septic source, e.g. teeth, ears, skin marks, e.g. rashes, café-au-lait spots, angiomata anterior fontanelle/head circumference in baby.

Central nervous system examination is described systematically from the head downwards and includes the following:

Cranial nerves 1-12 nerves.	**Conscious level and higher cerebral function** *Cognitive skills Memory Reasoning Emotional states.*	**Upper and lower limbs.** *Motor system*-wasting/tone/power *Sensory system*-pain/touch/temperature/proprioception/Stereognosis *Reflexes* *Co-ordination.*	**Trunk.** *sensation* *Reflexes*	**sphincters**

CRANIAL NERVE FUNTION AND ASSESSMENT

Note: to be completed on the 12 cranial nerves

Nerve's Name	*System*	*Function*	*Method of Assessment*
1 Olfactory	Sensory	Sense of smell	Ask patient to identify different nonirritating aromas such as coffee powder.
2 Optic	Sensory	Vision	Use Snellen chart: Ask the patient to read printed material.
3 Oculomotor	Motor	Extraocular Eye movement Pupil constriction and dilation.	• Assess direction of gaze • Measure pupil reaction to 7light reflex
4 Trochlear	Motor	Upward and downward movement of the eyeball	Assess direction of gaze
5 Trigeminal	Sensory and motor	Sensory nerve to skin of face	Motor nerve to muscles of jaw. Assess corneal reflex measure sensation of light, pain and touch across skin of face.Assess patient's ability to clench teeth.
6 Abducens	Motor	Lateral movements of eyeballs	Assess direction of gaze
7 Facial	Sensory and motor	Facial expression	Ask patient to smile, frown, puff out cheeks, raise and lower eye brows
8 Auditory	Sensory	Hearing	Assess patient's ability to hear spoken word.
9 Glosso-pharyngeal	Sensory and motor	Taste ability to swallow	Movement of tongue. Ask patient to identify sour, salty or sweet taste on back of tongue. Use tongue blade to

Contd...

Contd...

Nerve's Name	*System*	*Function*	*Method of Assessment*
			elicit gag reflex. Ask patient to move the tongue.
10 Vagus	Sensory and motor	Sensation of pharynx .	Ability to swallow. Movement of vocal cords. Ask patient to say "ah" observe movement of palate and pharynx.Use tongue bade to elicit gag reflex.Ask patient's speech for hoarseness.
11 Spinal accessory	Motor	Movement of head and shoulders.	Ask patient to shrug shoulders and turn head against examiner's passive resistance.
12 Hypo-glossal	Motor	Position of midline.	Ask patient to stick to tongue.

Conscious Level Assessment

Action	*Response*	*Score*
Eyes Open	Spontaneously To speech To pain None	4 3 2 1
Best Verbal Response	Oriented Confused Inappropriate words Incomprehensive sounds	5 4 3 2
Best Motor Response	obeys commands localized pain flexion withdrawal abnormal flexion abnormal extension flaccid	6 5 4 3 2 1
Total		15

A. COGNITIVE SKILL

1. Dominant Hemisphere Disorders

Listen to language pattern – Hesitant – Fluent	Expressive dysphasia Receptive dysphasia.
Does the patient understand simple/complex Spoken commands? e.g 'hold up both arms, touch the right ear with the left fifth finger.'	Receptive dysphasia.
Ask the patient to name the objects.	Normal dysphasia.
Does the patient read correctly?	Dyslexia
Does the patient write correctly?	Dysgraphia
Ask the patient to perform a numerical calculation, e.g. serial 7 test, where 7 is subtracted serially from 100	Dyscalculia
Can the patient recognize objects? e.g. ask the patient to select an object from a group.	Agnosia

2. Non-dominant Hemisphere Disorders

Note patient's ability to find his way around the ward or his home.	Geographical agnosia
Can the patient dress himself? Dressing apraxia	
Note the patient's ability to copy a geometric pattern, e.g. ask the patient to form a star with matches or copy a drawing of the cube.	Constructional apraxia

B. MEMORY SKILL

Testing requires alertness and is not possible in a confused or dysphasic patient.

- Immediate memory : Digit span—ask patient to repeat a sequence of 5, 6 or 7 random Numbers.
- Recent memory : Ask patient to describe present illness, duration of hospital stay.
  Or recent events in the news.
- Remote memory : Ask about events and circumstances occurring more than 5 years.
  Previously.

- Verbal memory : Ask patient to remember a sentence or a short story and test after 15 minutes.
- Visual memory : Ask patient to remember objects on a tray and test after 15 mints.

C. REASONING AND PROBLEM SOLVING SKILL

Test the patient with two-step calculations, e.g. 'I wish to buy 12 articles at 7 pence each. How much change will I receive from shop?

Ask patient to reverse 3 or 4 random numbers.

Ask patient to explain proverbs.

The examiner must compare patient's present reasoning ability with expected abilities based on job history and/or school work.

D. EMOTIONAL STATE

Note:
- Anxiety or excitement
- Depression or apathy
- Emotional behavior
- Uninhibited behavior
- Slowness of movement or responses.

UPPER AND LOWER LIMBS ASSESSMENT OF SENSORY NERVE FUNCTION

Sensory Function	*Equipment*	*Method*
Pain	Safety pin	Ask patient to tell you when dull or sharp sensation is felt. Alternately apply pointed and blunt ends of pin to skin's surface. Note areas of numbness or increased sensitivity.
Temperature	Two tests: • Tube filled with hot water, and • Tube filled with cold water	Touch patient's skin with tube.Ask client to identify hot/cold sensation.
Light Touch	Cotton ball or cotton tip applicator.	Apply light wisp of cotton to different points along skin surface. Ask patient to tell you when sensation is felt.

Contd...

Contd...

Sensory Function	*Equipment*	*Method*
Vibration	Tuning fork	Apply vibrating fork to distal inter-phalageal joint of great toe.
Position		Grasp patient's finger, holding it by its sides with your thumb and index finger. Alternate moving finger up and down. Ask patient to tell you whether finger is up or down. Repeat procedure with toes.
Two-point Discrimination	Two safety pins	Lightly apply points of two safety pins simultaneously to skin's surface. Ask if patient feels one or two pinpricks.

MOTOR SYSTEM—UPPER LIMBS

Appearance—Asymmetry or deformity
Muscle wasting
Muscle hypertrophy
Muscle fasciculation.

Tone—Try to relax the patient and alternately flex and extend the knee joint. Note the resistance.

Power—When testing each muscle group, think of root and nerve supply.

Test	*Nerve*	*Method*
Test for Serratus Anterior	C5, C6, C7 roots long thoracic nerve	Patient presses arms against wall Look for winging of scapula
Shoulder Abduction	Deltoid: C5, C6 roots axillary nerve.	Arm (at more than 15" from the vertical). Abducts against resistance.
Elbow Flexion	Biceps: C5, C6, roots musculocutaneous nerve. Brachioradialis: C5, C6 roots Radial nerve	Arm flexed against resistance with the hand fully supinated. Arm flexed against resistance with hand in mid-position between pronation and supination
Elbow Extension Finger Extension	Triceps: C6, C7, C8 roots Radial nerve Extensor digitorum: C7, C8 roots posterior inter-osseous nerve.	Patients extends arm against resistance. Patients extends fingers against resistance.

Contd...

Contd...

Test	*Nerve*	*Method*
Thumb Extension-Terminal Phalanx	Extensor pollicis longus and brevis: C7, C8 roots posterior inter-osseous nerve.	Thumb is extended against resistance.
Finger Flexion-Terminal Phalanx	Flexor digitorum profundus I and II: C7, C8 roots median nerve. Flexor digitorum profundus III and IV: C7, C8 roots ulnar nerve.	Examiner tries to extend patient's flexed terminal phalanges.
Thumb Opposition	Opponens pollicis: C8, T1 roots, median nerve.	Patient tries to touch the base of the 5 th finger with thumb against resistance.
Finger Abduction	1st dorsal interosseus: C8, T1 roots, ulnar nerve. Abductor digiti minimi: C8, T1 roots. Ulnar nerve.	Fingers abducted against resistance.

MOTOR SYSTEM—LOWER LIMBS

Appearance—Asymmetry or deformity.

- Muscle wasting
- Muscle hypertrophy
- Muscle fasciculation.

Tone—Try to relax the patient and alternately flex and extend the knee joint. Note the resistance.

Power—When testing each muscle group, think of root and nerve supply.

Test	*Nerve*	*Method*
Hip Flexion	llio-psoas: L1, L2, L3 roots. Femoral nerve.	Hip flexed against resistance.
Hip Extension	Gluteus maximus: L5, S1, S2 roots. inferior gluteal nerve.	Patient attempts to keep heel on bed against resistance.
Hip Abduction	Gluteus medius and minimus and tensor fasciae latae: L4, L5, S1 roots. Superior gluteal nerve	Patient lying on back tries to abduct the leg against resistance.

Contd...

Contd...

Test	*Nerve*	*Method*
Hip Adduction	Adductors:L2, L3, L4 roots. Obturator nerve.	Patient lying on back tries to pull knees together against resistance.
Knee Flexion	Hamstrings: L5, S1, S2 roots. Sciatic nerve	Patient pulls heel towards the buttock and tries to maintain this position against resistance.
Knee Extension	Quadriceps: L2, L3, L4 roots. Femoral nerve	Patient tries to extend knee against resistance.
Dorsi Flexion	Tibialis anterior: L4, L5 roots. Deep peroneal nerve.	Patient dorsiflexes the ankle against resistance. May have difficulty in walking on heels.
Plantar Flexion	Gastrocnemius, soleus: S1, S2 roots. Tibial nerve.	Patient plantarflexes the ankle against resistance. May have difficulty in walking on toes before weakness can be directly detected.
Toe Extension	Extensor hallucis longus, extensor digitorum longus:L5, S1 roots. Deep potoneal nerve.	Patient dorsiflexes the toes against resistance.
Inversion	Tibialis postorior L4, L5 root. Tibial nerve.	Patient inverts foot against resistance.
Eversion	Peroneous longus and bravis: L5, S1 roots. Superficial peroneal nerve.	Patient everts foot against resistancess

ASSESSMENT OF REFLEXES:

Deep Tendon Reflexes

Type	*Procedure*	*Normal Reflex*
Biceps	Flex patient's arm at the elbow with palms down. Place your thumb in the cubital fossa at base of the biceps tendon. Strike thumb with the reflex hammer.	Flexion of arm at elbow.

Contd...

Contd...

Type	*Procedure*	*Normal Reflex*
Triceps	Flex patient's elbow holding arm across the chest or hold upper arm horizontally and allow lower arm to go limp. Strike the triceps tendon just above the elbow.	Extension at elbow.
Patellar	Have patient sit with legs hanging freely over side of the bed or chair or have patient lie supine and support the knee in a flexed position. Briskly tap the patellar tendon just below the patella.	Extension of lower leg at knee.
Plantar	Have patient lie supine with legs straight and feet relaxed. Take handle end of the reflex hammer and stroke the lateral aspect of the sole from the heel to the ball of the foot curving across the ball.	Flexion of toes.

Trunk

Sensation Reflexes

Test pin prick and touch in dermatome distribution as for the upper limb.

Levels to remember: T5-at nipple
T10-at umbilicus
T12-at inguinal ligament.

Abdominal reflexes: T7-T12 roots. Stroke or lightly scratch the skin towards the umbilicus in each quadrant in turn. look for abdominal muscle contraction.

Sphincters

Examine abdomen for distended bladder.

Note evidence of urinary or faecal incontinence.

Anal reflex: S4, S5 roots.

A scratch on the skin bedside, the anus causes a reflex contraction of the anal sphincter.

PROCESS RECORDING

Definition

Process recording is a written account or verbatim recording of all that transpired immediately before, during and immediately following the nurse-patient interaction.

Purpose

- Assist to plan, structure and evaluate the interaction.
- Gain competency in interpreting and syntherizing raw data.
- Apply theory into practice.
- Increased awareness of her habitual, verbal and nonverbal communication patterns.
- Identify thoughts and feelings.
- Increase observation skills.
- Ability to identify problems and gain skills in solving them.

Uses

- Educative tool.
- Teaching tool.
- Diagnostic tool.
- Therapeutic tool.
- Pre-requisite for nursing process.

Pre-requisite for process recording

- Physical setting.
- Getting consent of the patient for the possibility of cassette recording.
- Confidentiality.

Procedure

- Introductory material.
  - Short description of the patient [name, age, sex, ect.]
  - Date, time, and place.
  - Thoughts and feelings.
  - Duration.
- Objectives—Short term goal and long-term goal.
- Record of interaction between nurse and the patient.
  - Verbal response.
  - Non verbal response.
  - Self evaluation.

- Analysis of the interaction.
  - Interpretation of the verbal and non verbal responses.
  - Thoughts and feelings.
  - Communication techniques.
  - Total time 30 mints. [Active time 20 mints and 10 mints for conclusion.]

VERBATUM

Name:

Age:

Sex:

Place:

Date and time:

Situation:

Day of admission:

Objectives of the interview:

1)

2)

3)

Nurse Verbal Response	*Nurse Non Verbal Response*	*Patient Verbal Response*	*Patient Non Verbal Response*	*Inference*

Conclusion:

Summary:

Chapter 2

ADMINISTRATION OF PSYCHOTHERAPEUTIC DRUGS

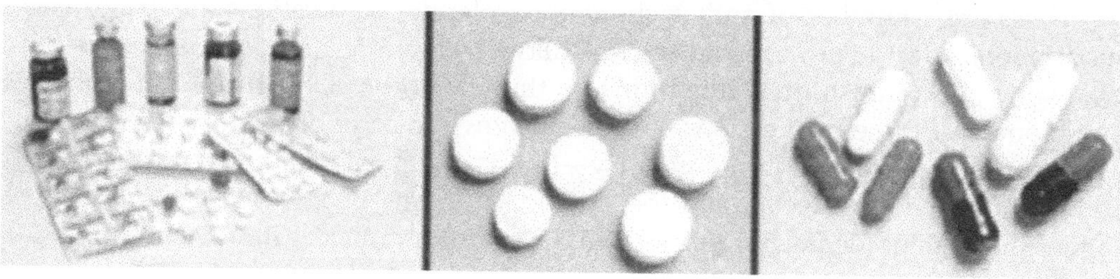

ANTIPSYCHOTIC DRUGS

INTRODUCTION

Medications for mental illnesses were first introduced in the early 1950s with the antipsychotic chlorpromazine. Other medications have followed. These medications have changed the lives of people with these disorders for the better.

Psychotherapeutic medications also may make other kinds of treatment more effective. Someone who is too depressed to talk, for instance, may have difficulty communicating during psychotherapy or counseling, but the right medication may improve symptoms so the person can respond. For many patients, a combination of psychotherapy and medication can be an effective method of treatment.

Questions for Your Doctor

The patient or a family member ask the following questions when a medication is prescribed:

- What is the name of the medication, and what is it supposed to do?
- How and when do I take it, and when do I stop taking it?
- What foods, drinks, or other medications should I avoid while taking the prescribed medication?
- Should it be taken with food or on an empty stomach?
- Is it safe to drink alcohol while on this medication?
- What are the side effects, and what should I do if they occur?

ANTIPSYCHOTIC MEDICATIONS

A person who is psychotic is out of touch with reality. People with psychosis may hear "voices" or have strange and illogical ideas (for example, thinking that others can hear their thoughts, or are trying to harm them, or that they are the President of the United States or some other famous person). They may get excited or angry for no apparent reason, or spend a lot of time by themselves, or in bed, sleeping during the day and staying awake at night. The person may neglect appearance, not bathing or changing clothes, and may be hard to talk to—barely talking or saying things that make no sense. They often are initially unaware that their condition is an illness.

There are a number of antipsychotic (neuroleptic) medications available. These medications affect neurotransmitters that allow communication between nerve cells. One such neurotransmitter, dopamine, is thought to be relevant to schizophrenia symptoms. All these medications have been shown to be effective for schizophrenia. The main differences are in the potency—that is, the dosage (amount) prescribed to produce therapeutic effects—and the side effects. Some people might think that the higher the dose of medication prescribed, the more serious the illness; but this is not always true.

The 1990s saw the development of several new drugs for schizophrenia, called "**atypical antipsychotics**." Because they have fewer side effects than the older drugs, today they are often used as a first-line treatment. The first atypical antipsychotic, clozapine (*Clozaril*), was introduced in the United States in 1990. In clinical trials, this medication was found to be more effective than conventional or "typical" antipsychotic medications in individuals with treatment - resistant schizophrenia (schizophrenia that has not responded to other drugs), and the risk of tardive dyskinesia (a movement disorder) was lower. However, because of the potential side effect of a serious blood disorder—agranulocytosis (loss of the white blood cells that fight infection)—patients who are on clozapine must have a blood test every 1 or 2 weeks. The inconvenience and cost of blood tests and the medication itself have made maintenance on clozapine difficult for many people. Clozapine, however, continues to be the drug of choice for treatment - resistant schizophrenia patients.

Several other atypical antipsychotics have been developed since clozapine was introduced. The first was risperidone (*Risperdal*), followed by olanzapine (*Zyprexa*), quetiapine (*Seroquel*), and ziprasidone (*Geodon*). Each has a unique side effect profile, but in general, these medications are better tolerated than the earlier drugs.

All these medications have their place in the treatment of schizophrenia, and doctors will choose among them. They will consider the person's symptoms, age, weight, and personal and family medication history.

Dosages and Side Effects

Most side effects of antipsychotic medications are mild. Many common ones lessen or disappear after the first few weeks of treatment. These include drowsiness, rapid heartbeat, and dizziness, when changing position.

Some people gain weight while taking medications and need to pay extra attention to diet and exercise to control their weight. Other side effects may include a decrease in sexual ability or interest, problems with menstrual periods, sunburn, or skin rashes. If a side effect occurs, the doctor should be told. He or she may prescribe a different medication, change the dosage or schedule, or prescribe an additional medication to control the side effects.

ANTIMANIC MEDICATIONS

Bipolar disorder is characterized by cycling mood changes: severe highs (mania) and lows (depression). Episodes may be predominantly manic or depressive, with normal mood between episodes. Mood swings may follow each other very closely, within days (rapid cycling), or may be separated by months to years. The "highs" and "lows" may vary in intensity and severity and can co-exist in "mixed" episodes.

Lithium

The medication used most often to treat bipolar disorder is lithium. Lithium evens out mood swings in both directions—From mania to depression, and depression to mania—So it is used not just for manic attacks or flare-ups of the illness but also as an ongoing maintenance treatment for bipolar disorder.

Although lithium will reduce severe manic symptoms in about 5 to 14 days, it may be weeks to several months before the condition is fully controlled. Antipsychotic medications are sometimes used in the first several days of treatment to control manic symptoms until the lithium begins to take effect. Antidepressants may also be added to lithium during the depressive phase of bipolar disorder. If given in the absence of lithium or another mood stabilizer, antidepressants may provoke a switch into mania in people with bipolar disorder.

Regular blood tests are an important part of treatment with lithium. If too little is taken, lithium will not be effective. If too much is taken, a variety of side effects may occur. The range between an effective dose and a toxic one is small. Blood lithium levels are checked at the beginning of treatment to determine the best lithium dosage. Once a person is stable and on a maintenance dosage, the lithium level should be checked every few months. How much lithium people need to take may vary over time, depending on how ill they are, their body chemistry, and their physical condition.

Side Effects of Lithium

When people first take lithium, they may experience side effects such as drowsiness, weakness, nausea, fatigue, hand tremor, or increased thirst and urination. Some may disappear or decrease quickly, although hand tremor may persist. Weight gain may also occur. Dieting will help, but crash diets should be avoided because they may raise or lower the lithium level. Drinking low-calorie or no-calorie beverages, especially water, will help keep weight down. Kidney changes—increased urination and, in children, enuresis (bed wetting)—may develop during treatment. These changes are generally manageable and are reduced by lowering the dosage. Because lithium may cause the thyroid gland to become underactive (hypothyroidism) or sometimes enlarged (goiter), thyroid function monitoring is a part of the therapy. To restore normal thyroid function, thyroid hormone may be given along with lithium.

ANTICONVULSANTS

The anticonvulsant valproic acid (*Depakote, divalproex sodium*) is the main alternative therapy for bipolar disorder. It is as effective in non-rapid-cycling bipolar disorder as lithium and appears to be superior to lithium in rapid-cycling bipolar disorder. Although valproic acid can cause gastrointestinal side effects, the incidence is low. Other adverse effects occasionally reported are headache, double vision, dizziness, anxiety, or confusion. Because in some cases valproic acid has caused liver dysfunction, liver function tests should be performed before therapy and at frequent intervals, thereafter, particularly during the first 6 months of therapy.

Other anticonvulsants used for bipolar disorder include carbamazepine (*Tegretol*), lamotrigine (*Lamictal*), gabapentin (*Neurontin*), and topiramate (*Topamax*). The evidence for anticonvulsant effectiveness is stronger for acute mania than for long-term maintenance of bipolar disorder.

ANTIDEPRESSANT MEDICATIONS

Depressed people will seem "sad", or "down," or may be unable to enjoy their normal activities. They may have no appetite and lose weight (although some people eat more and gain weight when depressed). They may sleep too much or too little, have difficulty going to sleep, sleep restlessly, or awaken very early in the morning. They may speak of feeling guilty, worthless, or hopeless; they may lack energy or be jumpy and agitated. They may think about killing themselves and may even make a suicide attempt. Some depressed people have delusions (false, fixed ideas) about poverty, sickness, or sinfulness that are related to their depression. Often feelings of depression are worse at a particular time of day, for instance, every morning or every evening.

Not everyone who is depressed has all these symptoms, but everyone who is depressed has at least some of them, co-existing, on most days. Depression can range in intensity from mild to severe. Depression can co-occur with other medical disorders such as cancer, heart disease, stroke, Parkinson's disease, Alzheimer's disease, and diabetes. In such cases, the depression is often overlooked and is not treated. If the depression is recognized and treated, a person's quality of life can be greatly improved.

Antidepressants are used most often for serious depressions, but they can also be helpful for some milder depressions. Antidepressants are not "uppers" or stimulants, but rather take away or reduce the symptoms of depression and help depressed people feel the way they did before they became depressed.

Early Antidepressants. From the 1960s through the 1980s, **tricyclic antidepressants** (named for their chemical structure) were the first line of treatment for major depression. Most of these medications affected two chemical neurotransmitters, norepinephrine and serotonin. Though the tricyclics are as effective in treating depression as the newer antidepressants, their side effects are usually more unpleasant; thus, today tricyclics such as imipramine, amitriptyline, nortriptyline, and desipramine are used as a second- or third-line treatment. Other antidepressants introduced during this period were **monoamine oxidase inhibitors (MAOIs)**. MAOIs are effective for some people with major depression who do not respond to other antidepressants. They are also effective for the treatment of panic disorder and bipolar depression. MAOIs approved for the treatment of depression are phenelzine (Nardil), tranylcypromine (Parnate), and isocarboxazid (Marplan). Because substances in certain foods, beverages, and medications can cause dangerous interactions when combined with MAOIs, people on these agents must adhere to dietary restrictions. This has deterred many clinicians and patients from using these effective medications, which are in fact quite safe when used as directed.

The past decade has seen the introduction of many new antidepressants that work as well as the older ones but have fewer side effects. Some of these medications primarily affect one neurotransmitter, serotonin, and are called **selective serotonin reuptake inhibitors (SSRIs)**. These include fluoxetine (*Prozac*), sertraline (*Zoloft*), fluvoxamine (*Luvox*), paroxetine (*Paxil*), and citalopram (*Celexa*).

The late 1990s ushered in new medications that, like the tricyclics, affect both norepinephrine and serotonin but have fewer side effects. These new medications include venlafaxine (*Effexor*) and nefazadone (*Serzone*).

Side Effects of Antidepressant Medications

Antidepressants may cause mild, and often temporary, side effects (sometimes referred to as adverse effects) in some people. Typically, these are not serious. However, any reactions or side effects that are unusual, annoying, or that interfere with functioning should be reported to the doctor immediately. The most common side effects of tricyclic antidepressants, and ways to deal with them, are as follows:

- *Dry mouth*—It is helpful to drink sips of water; chew sugarless gum; brush teeth daily.
- *Constipation*—Bran cereals, prunes, fruit, and vegetables should be in the diet.
- *Bladder problems*—Emptying the bladder completely may be difficult, and the urine stream may not be as strong as usual. Older men with enlarged prostate conditions may be at particular risk for this problem. The doctor should be notified if there is any pain.
- *Sexual problems*—Sexual functioning may be impaired; if this is worrisome, it should be discussed with the doctor.

- *Blurred vision*—This is usually temporary and will not necessitate new glasses. Glaucoma patients should report any change in vision to the doctor.
- *Dizziness*—Rising from the bed or chair slowly is helpful.
- *Drowsiness as a daytime problem*—This usually passes soon. A person who feels drowsy or sedated should not drive or operate heavy equipment. The more sedating antidepressants are generally taken at bedtime to help sleep and to minimize daytime drowsiness.
- *Increased heart rate*—Pulse rate is often elevated. Older patients should have an electrocardiogram (ECG) before beginning tricyclic treatment.
  The newer antidepressants, including SSRIs, have different types of side effects, as follows:
- *Sexual problems*—Fairly common, but reversible, in both men and women. The doctor should be consulted if the problem is persistent or worrisome.
- *Headache*—This will usually go away after a short time.
- *Nausea*—May occur after a dose, but it will disappear quickly.
- *Nervousness and insomnia (trouble falling asleep or waking often during the night)*—These may occur during the first few weeks; dosage reductions or time will usually resolve them.
- *Agitation (feeling jittery)*—If this happens for the first time after the drug is taken and is more than temporary, the doctor should be notified.

Any of these side effects may be amplified when an SSRI is combined with other medications that affect serotonin. In the most extreme cases, such a combination of medications (e.g., an SSRI and an MAOI) may result in a potentially serious or even fatal "serotonin syndrome," characterized by fever, confusion, muscle rigidity, and cardiac, liver, or kidney problems.

ANTIANXIETY MEDICATIONS

Anxiety is often manageable and mild, but sometimes it can present serious problems. A high level or prolonged state of anxiety can make the activities of daily life difficult or impossible. People may have generalized anxiety disorder (GAD) or more specific anxiety disorders such as panic, phobias, obsessive-compulsive disorder (OCD), or post-traumatic stress disorder (PTSD).

Both antidepressants and antianxiety medications are used to treat anxiety disorders. The broad-spectrum activity of most antidepressants provides effectiveness in anxiety disorders as well as depression. The first medication specifically approved for use in the treatment of OCD was the tricyclic antidepressant clomipramine (*Anafranil*). The SSRIs, fluoxetine (*Prozac*), fluvoxamine (*Luvox*), paroxetine (*Paxil*), and sertraline (*Zoloft*) have now been approved for use with OCD. Paroxetine has also been approved for social anxiety disorder (social phobia), GAD, and panic disorder; and sertraline is approved for panic disorder and PTSD. Venlafaxine (*Effexor*) has been approved for GAD.

Antianxiety medications include the benzodiazepines, which can relieve symptoms within a short time. They have relatively few side effects: drowsiness and loss of coordination are most common; fatigue and mental slowing or confusion can also occur. These effects make it dangerous for people taking benzodiazepines to drive or operate some machinery. Other side effects are rare.

The only medication specifically for anxiety disorders other than the benzodiazepines is buspirone (*BuSpar*). Unlike the benzodiazepines, buspirone must be taken consistently for at least 2 weeks to achieve an antianxiety effect and therefore cannot be used on an "as-needed" basis.

Beta blockers, medications often used to treat heart conditions and high blood pressure, are sometimes used to control "performance anxiety" when the individual must face a specific stressful situation—a speech, a presentation in class, or an important meeting. Propranolol (*Inderal, Inderide*) is a commonly used beta blocker.

MEDICATIONS FOR SPECIAL GROUPS

Children, the elderly, and pregnant and nursing women have special concerns and needs when taking psychotherapeutic medications. Some effects of medications on the growing body, the aging body, and the childbearing body are known, but much remains to be learned. Research in these areas is ongoing.

Children

Many treatments are available to help these children. The treatments include both medications and psychotherapy—behavioral therapy, treatment of impaired social skills, parental and family therapy, and group therapy. The therapy used is based on the child's diagnosis and individual needs.

When the decision is reached that a child should take medication, active monitoring by all caretakers (parents, teachers, and others who have charge of the child) is essential. Children should be watched and questioned for side effects because many children, especially younger ones, do not volunteer information. They should also be monitored to see that they are actually taking the medication and taking the proper dosage on the correct schedule.

Childhood-onset depression and anxiety are increasingly recognized and treated. However, the best - known and most treated childhood onset mental disorder is attention deficit hyperactivity disorder (ADHD). Children with ADHD exhibit symptoms such as short attention span, excessive motor activity, and impulsivity which interfere with their ability to function especially at school. The medications most commonly prescribed for ADHD are called stimulants. These include methylphenidate (*Ritalin, Metadate, Concerta*), amphetamine (*Adderall*), dextroamphetamine (*Dexedrine, Dextrostat*), and pemoline (*Cylert*). Because of its potential for serious side effects on the liver, pemoline is not ordinarily used as a first-line therapy for ADHD.

Some antidepressants such as bupropion (*Wellbutrin*) are often used as alternative medications for ADHD for children who do not respond to or tolerate stimulants.

Elderly

Persons over the age of 65 make up almost 13 percent of the population of the United States, but they receive 30 percent of prescriptions filled. The elderly generally have more medical problems, and many of them are taking medications for more than one of these conditions. In addition, they tend to be more sensitive to medications. Even healthy older people eliminate some medications from the body more slowly than younger persons and therefore require a lower or less frequent dosage to maintain an effective level of medication.

The elderly are also more likely to take too much of a medication accidentally because they forget that they have taken a dose and take another one. The use of a 7-day pill-box, as described earlier in this brochure, can be especially helpful for an elderly person.

The elderly and those close to them—friends, relatives, caretakers—need to pay special attention and watch for adverse (negative) physical and psychological responses to medication. Because they often take more medications—not only those prescribed but also over-the-counter preparations and home, folk, or herbal remedies—the possibility of adverse drug interactions is high.

Women during the Childbearing Years

Because there is a risk of birth defects with some psychotropic medications during early pregnancy, a woman who is taking such medication and wishes to become pregnant should discuss her plans with her doctor. In general, it is desirable to minimize or avoid the use of medication during early pregnancy. If a woman on medication discovers that she is pregnant, she should contact her doctor immediately. She and the doctor can decide how best to handle her therapy during and following the pregnancy. Some precautions that should be taken are:

- If possible, lithium should be discontinued during the first trimester (first 3 months of pregnancy) because of an increased risk of birth defects.
- If the patient has been taking an anticonvulsant such as carbamazepine (*Tegretol*) or valproic acid (*Depakote*)—both of which have a somewhat higher risk than lithium—an alternate treatment should be used if at all possible. The risks of two other anticonvulsants, lamotrigine (*Lamictal*) and gabapentin (*Neurontin*) are unknown. An alternative medication for any of the anticonvulsants might be a conventional antipsychotic or an antidepressant, usually an SSRI. If essential to the patient's health, an anticonvulsant should be given at the lowest dose possible. It is especially important when taking an anticonvulsant to take a recommended dosage of folic acid during the first trimester.

- Benzodiazepines are not recommended during the first trimester.

The decision to use a psychotropic medication should be made only after a careful discussion between the woman, her partner, and her doctor about the risks and benefits to her and the baby. If, after discussion, they agree it, best to continue medication, the lowest effective dosage should be used, or the medication can be changed. For a woman with an anxiety disorder, a change from a benzodiazepine to an antidepressant might be considered. Cognitive-behavioral therapy may be beneficial in helping an anxious or depressed person to lower medication requirements. For women with severe mood disorders, a course of electroconvulsive therapy (ECT) is sometimes recommended during pregnancy as a means of minimizing exposure to riskier treatments.

After the baby is born, there are other considerations. Women with bipolar disorder are at particularly high risk for a postpartum episode. If they have stopped medication during pregnancy, they may want to resume their medication just prior to delivery or shortly thereafter. They will also need to be especially careful to maintain their normal sleep-wake cycle. Women who have histories of depression should be checked for recurrent depression or postpartum depression during the months after the birth of a child.

Women who are planning to breastfeed should be aware that small amounts of medication pass into the breast milk. In some cases, steps can be taken to reduce the exposure of the nursing infant to the mother's medication, for instance, by timing doses to post-feeding sleep periods. The potential benefits and risks of breastfeeding by a woman taking psychotropic medication should be discussed and carefully weighed by the patient and her physician.

A woman who is taking birth control pills should be sure that her doctor knows this. The estrogen in these pills may affect the breakdown of medications by the body—for example, increasing side effects of some anti–anxiety medications or reducing their ability to relieve symptoms of anxiety. Also, some medications, including carbamazepine and some antibiotics, and an herbal supplement, St. John's wort, can cause an oral contraceptive to be ineffective.

Chapter 3

APPLICATION OF PSYCHIATRIC NURSING PROCESS

MULTI-AXIAL SYSTEM

The DSM-IV organizes each psychiatric diagnosis into five levels (axes) relating to different aspects of disorder or disability:

- *Axis I:* Clinical disorders, including major mental disorders, as well as developmental and learning disorders
- *Axis II:* Underlying pervasive or personality conditions, as well as mental retardation
- *Axis III:* Acute medical conditions and physical disorders.
- *Axis IV:* Psychosocial and environmental factors contributing to the disorder
- *Axis V:* Global Assessment of Functioning or Children's Global Assessment Scale for children under the age of 18 (on a scale from 100 to 1).

Common Axis I disorders include depression, anxiety disorders, bipolar disorder, ADHD, phobias, and schizophrenia.

Common Axis II disorders include personality disorders: paranoid personality disorder, schizoid personality disorder, schizotypal personality disorder, borderline personality disorder, antisocial personality disorder, narcissistic personality disorder, histrionic personality disorder, avoidant personality disorder, dependent personality disorder, obsessive-compulsive personality disorder, and mental retardation.

Common Axis III disorders include brain injuries and other medical/physical disorders which may aggravate existing diseases or present symptoms similar to other disorders.

The Global Assessment of Functioning (GAF) is a numeric scale (0 through 100) used by mental health clinicians and physicians to subjectively rate the social, occupational and psychological functioning of adults, e.g., how well or adaptively one is meeting various problems in living. The scale is presented and described in the DSM-IV-TR.

Children and adolescents under the age of 18 are evaluated on the Children's Global Assessment Scale, or C-GAS:

91-100: Superior functioning in a wide range of activities, life's problems never seem to get out of hand, is sought out by others because of his or her many qualities. No symptoms.

81-90: Absent or minimal symptoms, good functioning in all areas, interested and involved in a wide range of activities, socially effective, generally satisfied with life, no more than everyday problems or concerns.

71-80: If symptoms are present they are transient and expectable reactions to psychosocial stresses; no more than slight impairment in social, occupational, or school functioning.

61-70: Some mild symptoms OR some difficulty in social, occupational, or school functioning, but generally functioning pretty well, has some meaningful interpersonal relationships.

51-60: Moderate symptoms OR any moderate difficulty in social, occupational, or school functioning.

41-50: Serious symptoms OR any serious impairment in social, occupational, or school functioning.

31-40: Some impairment in reality testing or communication OR major impairment in several areas, such as work or school, family relations, judgment, thinking, or mood.

21-30: Behavior is considerably influenced by delusions or hallucinations OR serious impairment in communications or judgment OR inability to function in all areas.

11-20: Some danger of hurting self or others OR occasionally fails to maintain minimal personal hygiene OR gross impairment in communication.

1-10: Persistent danger of severely hurting self or others OR persistent inability to maintain minimum personal hygiene OR serious suicidal act with clear expectation of death.

0: Not enough information available to provide GAF.

PSYCHIATRIC NURSING CARE PLANS

1. General Care Plans

Building a Trust Relationship
Discharge Planning
Deficient Knowledge
Noncompliance
Supporting the Caregiver

2. Community-based Care

Persistent and Severe Mental Illness
Acute Episode Care
Partial Community Support

3. Disorders Diagnosed in Childhood or Adolescence

Attention-Deficit/Hyperactivity Disorder
Conduct Disorders
Adjustment Disorders of Adolescence

4. Delirium and Dementia

Delirium
Dementia

5. Substance-related Disorders

Alcohol Withdrawal
Substance Withdrawal
Dual Diagnosis

6. Schizophrenia and Psychotic Disorders/Symptoms

Schizophrenia
Delusions
Hallucinations
Delusional Disorder
Psychotic Behavior Related to a Medical Condition

7. Mood Disorders and Related Behaviors

Major Depressive Disorder
Suicidal Behavior
Bipolar Disorder, Manic Episode

8. Anxiety Disorders

Anxious Behavior
Phobias
Obsessive-Compulsive Disorder
Posttraumatic Stress Disorder

9. Somatoform and Dissociative Disorders

Somatization Disorder
Conversion Disorder

Hypochondriasis
Dissociative Disorders

10. Eating Disorders

Anorexia Nervosa
Bulimia Nervosa

11. Sleep Disorders and Adjustment Disorders

Sleep Disorders
Adjustment Disorders of Adults

12. Personality Disorders

Paranoid Personality Disorder
Schizoid and Schizotypal Personality Disorders
Antisocial Personality Disorder
Borderline Personality Disorder
Dependent Personality Disorder
Passive–Aggressive Personality Disorder

13. Behavioral and Problem-based Care Plans

Withdrawn Behavior
Hostile Behavior
Aggressive Behavior
Sexual, Emotional, or Physical Abuse

NANDA-APPROVED NURSING DIAGNOSES

This list represents the NANDjL-approved nursing diagnoses for clinical use and testing:
Activity Intolerance
Activity Intolerance, Risk for
Adjustment, Impaired
Airway Clearance, Ineffective
Allergy Response, Latex
Allergy Response, Risk for Latex
Anxiety
Anxiety, Death

Aspiration, Risk for
Attachment, Risk for Impaired Parent/Infant/Child
Autonomic Dysreflexia
Autonomic Dysreflexia, Risk for
Body Image, Disturbed
Body Temperature, Risk for Imbalanced
Bowel Incontinence
Breastfeeding, Effective
Breastfeeding, Ineffective
Breastfeeding, Interrupted
Breathing Pattern, Ineffective
Cardiac Output, Decreased
Caregiver Role Strain
Caregiver Role Strain, Risk for
Comfort, Impaired
Communication, Impaired Verbal
Conflict, Decisional
Conflict, Parental Role
Confusion, Acute
Confusion, Chronic
Constipation
Constipation, Perceived
Constipation, Risk for
Coping, Ineffective
Coping, Ineffective Community
Coping, Readiness for Enhanced Community
Coping, Defensive
Coping, Compromised Family
Coping, Disabled Family
Coping, Readiness for Enhanced Family
Denial, Ineffective
Dentition, Impaired
Development, Risk for Delayed
Diarrhea
Disuse Syndrome, Risk for
Diversional Activity, Deficient

Energy Field, Disturbed
Environmental Interpretation Syndrome, Impaired
Failure .to Thrive, Adult
Falls, Risk for
Family Processes: Alcoholism, Dysfunctional
Family Processes: Interrupted
Fatigue
Fear
Fluid Volume, Deficient
Fluid Volume, Excess
Fluid Volume, Risk for Deficient
Fluid Volume, Risk for Imbalanced
Gas Exchange, Impaired
Grieving
Grieving, Anticipatory
Grieving, Dysfunctional
Growth and Development, Delayed
Growth, Risk for Disproportionate
Health Maintenance, Risk for Ineffective
Health-Seeking Behaviors
Home Maintenance, Impaired
Hopelessness
Hyperthermia
Hypothermia
Identity, Disturbed Personal
Incontinence, Functional Urinary
Incontinence, Reflex Urinary
Incontinence, Risk for Urge Urinary
Incontinence, Stress Urinary
Incontinence, Total Urinary
Incontinence, Urge Urinary
Infant Behavior, Disorganized
Infant Behavior, Readiness for Enhanced Organized.
Infant Behavior, Risk for Disorganized
Infant Feeding Pattern, Ineffective
Infection, Risk for

Injury, Risk for
Injury, Risk for Perioperative-Positioning
Intracranial, Adaptive Capacity, Decreased
Knowledge, Deficient
Loneliness, Risk for
Memory, Impaired
Mobility, Impaired Bed
Mobility, Impaired Physical
Mobility, Impaired Wheelchair
Nausea
Neglect, Unilateral
Noncompliance
Nutrition: Less Than Body Requirements, Imbalanced
Nutrition: More Than Body Requirements, Imbalanced
Oral Mucous Membrane, Impaired
Pain, Acute
Pain, Chronic
Parenting, Impaired
Parenting, Risk for Imparled
Peripheral Neurovascular Dysfunction, Risk for
Poisoning, Risk for
Post-Trauma Syndrome
Post-Trauma Syndrome, Risk for
Powerlessness
Powerlessness, Risk for
Protection, Ineffective
Rape-Trauma Syndrome
Rape-Trauma Syndrome; Compound Reaction
Rape-Trauma Syndrome; Silent Reaction
Relocation Stress Syndrome
Relocation Stress Syndrome, Risk for
Role Performance, Ineffective
Self-Care Deficit
Self-Care Deficit, Bathing/Hygiene
Self-Care Deficit, Feeding
Self-Care Deficit, Toileting
Self-Esteem, Chronic Low

Self-Esteem, Situational Low
Self-Esteem, Risk for Situational Low
Self-Mutilation
Sensory Perception, Disturbed
Sexual Dysfunction
Sexuality Patterns, Ineffective
Skin Integrity, Impaired
Skin Integrity, Risk tor Impaired
Sleep Deprivation
Sleep Pattern, Disturbed
Social Interaction, Impaired
Social Isolation
Sorrow, Chronic
Spiritual Distress
Spiritual Distress, Risk for
Spiritual Well-Being, Readiness for Enhanced
Suffocation, Risk for
Suicide, Risk for
Surgical Recovery, Delayed
Swallowing, Impaired
Therapeutic Regimen Management, Effective
Therapeutic Regimen Management, Ineffective
Therapeutic Regimen Management, Ineffective Community
Therapeutic Regimen Management, Ineffective Family
Thermoregulation, Ineffective
Thought Processes, Disturbed
Tissue Perfusion, Ineffective
Transfer Ability, Impaired
Trauma, Risk for
Urinary Elimination, Impaired
Urinary Retention
Ventilation, Impaired Spontaneous
Ventilatory Weaning Response, Dysfunctional (DVWR)
Violence, Risk for Other-Directed
Violence, Risk for Self-Directed
Walking, Impaired

1. SCHIZOPHRENIA

Nursing Diagnosis	*Assessment Data*	*Expected Outcomes*
• Disturbed personal identity • Inability to distinguish between self and nonself	• Bizarre behavior • Regressive behavior • Loss of ego boundaries (inability to differentiate self from the external environment) • Disorientation • Disorganized, illogical thinking • Flat or inappropriate affect • Feelings of anxiety, fear, or agitation • Aggressive behavior toward others or property	• Be free from injury • Not harm others or destroy property • Establish contact with reality • Demonstrate or verbalize decreased psychotic symptoms and feelings of anxiety, agitation, and so forth Participate in the therapeutic milieu

NURSING INTERVENTIONS

- Reassure the client that the environment is safe by briefly and simply explaining routines, procedures, and so forth.
- Protect the client from harming himself or herself or others. Remove items that could be used in self-destructive behavior.
- Remove the client from the group if his or her behavior becomes too bizarre, disturbing, or dangerous to others.
- Help the client's group, accept the client's "strange" behavior. Give simple explanations to the client's group as needed (e.g., "[Client] is very sick right now; he [or she] needs our understanding and support.").
- Consider the other client's needs. Plan for at least one staff member to be available to other clients, if several staff members are needed to care for this client.
- Explain to other clients that they have not done anything to warrant the client's verbal or physical threats; rather, the threats are the result of the client's illness.
- Set limits on the client's behavior when he or she is unable to do so (when the behavior interferes with other clients or becomes destructive). Do not set limits to punish the client.
- Decrease excessive stimuli in the environment. The client may not respond favorably to gym activities, competitive activities, or activities in large groups if he or she is still actively psychotic.
- Be aware of PRN medications and the client's varying need for them.
- Reorient the client to person, place, and time as indicated (call the client by name, tell the client where he or she is, and so forth).

- Spend time with the client even when he or she is unable to respond verbally or in a coherent manner. Convey your interest and caring.
- Make only promises that you can realistically keep.
- Limit the client's environment to enhance his or her feelings of security.
- Help the client establish what is real and unreal. Validate the client's real perceptions, and correct the client's misperceptions in a matter-of-fact manner. Do not argue with the client, but do not give support for misperceptions.
- Stay with the client when he or she is frightened. Touching the client can sometimes be therapeutic. Evaluate the effectiveness of the use of touch with the client before using it consistently.
- Be simple, direct, and concise when speaking to the client.
- Talk with the client about simple, concrete things; avoid ideologic or theoretical discussions.
- Direct activities toward helping the client accept and remain in contact with reality.
- Initially, assign the same staff members to work with the client.
- Begin with one-to-one interactions, and then progress to small groups as tolerated (introduce slowly).
- Establish and maintain a daily routine; explain any variation in this routine to the client.
- Set realistic goals. Set daily goals and expectations.
- Make the client aware of your expectations for him or her.
- At first, do not offer choices to the client ("Would you like to go to activities?" "What would you like to eat?").
- Instead, approach the client in a directive manner ("It is time to eat. Please pick up your fork").
- Gradually, as the client can tolerate it, provide opportunities for him or her to accept responsibility and make personal decisions.

Nursing Diagnosis	*Assessment Data*	*Expected Outcomes*
Social Isolation Aloneness experienced by the individual and perceived as imposed by others and as a negative or threatening state.	• Inappropriate or inadequate emotional responses • Poor interpersonal relationships • Feeling threatened in social situations • Difficulty with verbal communication • Exaggerated responses to stimuli	• Report increased feelings of self-worth • Identify strengths and assets • Engage in social interaction

NURSING INTERVENTIONS

- Provide attention in a sincere, interested manner.
- Support any successes or responsibilities fulfilled, projects, interactions with staff members and other clients, and so forth.
- Avoid trying to convince the client verbally of his or her own worth.
- Teach the client social skills. Describe and demonstrate specific skills, such as eye contact, attentive listening, nodding, and so forth.
- Discuss the type of topics that are appropriate for casual social conversation, such as the weather, local events, news, and so forth.
- Help the client improve his or her grooming; assist when necessary in bathing, doing laundry, and so forth.
- Help the client accept as much responsibility for personal grooming as he or she can (do not do something for the client that he or she can do alone).

Nursing Diagnosis	*Assessment Data*	*Expected Outcomes*
• Bathing/Hygiene Self Care Deficit: • Impaired ability to perform or complete bathing/hygiene activities for oneself. • Dressing/Grooming self care deficit: • Impaired ability to perform or complete dressing and grooming activities for self. • Feeding self care deficit: • Impaired ability to perform or complete feeding activities. • Toileting self care deficit: • Impaired ability to perform or complete own toileting activities.	• Disturbance of self initiated, goal-directed activity • Poor personal hygiene • Inability to follow through with completion of daily tasks • Apathy Anergy, or inability to use energy productively	• Establish an adequate balance of rest, sleep, and activity • Establish nutritional eating patterns Participate in self care activities

NURSING INTERVENTIONS

- Be alert to the client's physical needs.
- Observe the client's pattern of food and fluid intake; you may need to monitor and record intake, output, and daily weight.

- Monitor the client's elimination patterns. You may need to use PRN medication to establish regularity.
- Explain any task in short, simple steps.
- Using clear, direct sentences, instruct the client to do one part of the task at a time.
- Tell the client your expectations directly. Do not ask the client to choose unnecessarily.
- Tell the client it is time to eat or get dressed rather than asking if he or she wants to eat or dress.
- Do not confuse the client with reasons as to why things are to be done.
- Allow the client ample time to complete any task.
- Remain with the client throughout the task; do not attempt to hurry the client.
- Assist the client as needed to maintain daily functions and adequate personal hygiene.
- Gradually withdraw assistance and supervise the client's grooming or other self-care skills.
- Raise the client for completed activities of daily living and for initiating self-care activities.

2. BIPOLAR DISORDER, MANIC EPISODE

Nursing Diagnosis	*Assessment Data*	*Expected Outcomes*
Risk for other-directed violence At risk for behaviors in which an individual demonstrates that he/she can be physically, emotionally, and/or sexually harmful to others.	• Restlessness • Hyperactivity • Agitation • Hostile behavior • Threatened or actual aggression toward self or others • Low self-esteem	• Demonstrate decreased restlessness, hyperactivity, and agitation • Demonstrate decreased hostility Not harm himself or herself or others

NURSING INTERVENTIONS

- Provide a safe environment for the client.
- Decrease environmental stimuli whenever possible.
- Respond to cues of increased restlessness or agitation by removing stimuli and perhaps isolating the client; a single or private occupancy room may be beneficial.
- Administer chemotherapy (probably lithium or antipsychotic medications initially). Use PRN medication judiciously, preferably before the client's behavior becomes destructive.
- Provide a consistent, structured environment. Let the client know what is expected of him or her. Set goals with the client as soon as possible.

- Give simple direct explanations for routine actions, procedures, tests, and so forth. Do not argue with the client.
- Encourage the client to verbalize feelings of anxiety, anger, or fear. Explore ways to relieve stress and tension with the client as soon as possible.
- Encourage supervised physical activity.

Nursing Diagnosis	*Assessment Data*	*Expected Outcomes*
Defensive Coping Repeated projection of falsely positive self-evaluation based on a self-protective pattern that defends against underlying perceived threats to positive self regard.	• Denial of problems • Exaggeration of achievements • Grandiose schemes, plans, or stated self-image • Buying sprees • Inappropriate, bizarre, or flamboyant dress or use of makeup or jewelry • Flirtatious, seductive behavior Sexual acting-out	Demonstrate increased feelings of self-worth Demonstrate more appropriate appearance (dress, use of makeup, and so forth)

NURSING INTERVENTIONS

- Ignore or withdraw your attention from bizarre appearance and behavior and sexual actingout, as much as possible.
- Initially, structure tasks at which the client will succeed (short-term, simple projects or responsibilities, occupational or recreational therapy activities).
- Gradually increase the number and complexity of activities and responsibilities expected of the client.
- Give feedback at each level of accomplishment.

Nursing Diagnosis	*Assessment Data*	*Expected Outcomes*
Disturbed Thought Processes Disruption in cognitive operations and activities.	• Disorientation • Decreased concentration, short attention span • Loose associations (loosely and poorly associated ideas) • Push of speech (rapid, forced speech) • Tangentiality of ideas and speech • Hallucinations Delusions	• Demonstrate orientation to person, place, and time • Demonstrate decreased hallucinations or delusions • Demonstrate an increased attention span • Talk with others about present reality • Demonstrate decreased push of speech, tangentiality, loose associations

NURSING INTERVENTIONS

- Initially, assign the client to the same staff members when possible (keep in mind the staff member's ability to work with a manic client for extended periods of time).
- Reorient the client to person, place, and time as indicated (call the client by name, tell the client your name, tell the client where he or she is and the date, and so forth).
- Spend time with the client.
- Show acceptance of the client as a person.
- Use a firm yet calm, relaxed approach.
- Make only promises you can realistically keep.
- Set and maintain limits on behavior that is destructive or adversely affects others.
- Decrease environmental stimuli whenever possible.
- Respond to cues of increased restlessness or agitation by removing stimuli and perhaps isolating the client; a single or private occupancy room may be beneficial.
- Limit group activities in terms of size of group and frequency of activities based on the client's level of tolerance.
- Provide a consistent, structured environment.
- Let the client know what is expected of him or her.
- Set goals with the client as soon as possible.
- Help the client plan activities within his or her scope of achievement.
- Avoid highly competitive activities.
- Evaluate how much stimuli and responsibility the client can tolerate with respect to group activities, interactions with others, or visitors, and attempt to limit these accordingly.
- Encourage the client's appropriate expression of feelings regarding future treatment plans or discharge plans.
- Support any realistic goals and plans the patient proposes.

Nursing Diagnosis	*Assessment Data*	*Expected Outcomes*
Deficient Knowledge (Specify) Absence or deficiency of cognitive information related to a specific topic.	• Inappropriate behavior related to self-care • Inadequate retention of information presented • Inadequate understanding of information presented	Participate in learning about his or her illness, treatment, and safe use of medications

NURSING INTERVENTIONS

- Teach the client and family or significant others about manic behavior, bipolar disorder, and other problems as indicated.

- Inform the client and family or significant others about chemotherapy: dosage, the need to take the medication only as prescribed, the toxic symptoms ,the need to monitor blood levels, and other considerations.
- Explain information in clear, simple terms. Reinforce teaching with written material as indicated.
- Ask the client and family or significant others to state their understanding of the material as you explain.
- Encourage the client to ask questions and to express feelings and concerns.
- Stress to the client and family or significant others that medications must be taken regularly and continually to be effective; just because the client feels better or because his or her mood is level, is not sufficient cause to discontinue the drug.

3. MAJOR DEPRESSIVES

Nursing Diagnosis	*Assessment Data*	*Expected Outcomes*
Ineffective Coping Inability to form a valid appraisal of the stressors, inadequate choices of practiced responses, and/or inability to use available resources.	• Suicidal ideas or behavior • Slowed mental processes • Disordered thoughts • Feelings of despair, hopelessness, and worthlessness • Guilt • Anhedonia (inability to experience pleasure) • Disorientation • Generalized restlessness or agitation • Sleep disturbances: early awakening, insomnia, or excessive sleeping • Anger or hostility (may not be overt) • Rumination • Delusions, hallucinations, or other psychotic symptoms • Sexual dysfunction: diminished interest in sexual activity, inability to experience pleasure • Fear of intensity of feelings • Anxiety	Be free from self-inflicted harm. Engage in reality-based interactions. Be oriented to person, place, and time. Express anger or hostility outwardly in a safe manner

NURSING INTERVENTIONS

- Provide a safe environment for the client.
- Continually assess the client's potential for suicide.
- Observe the client closely, especially under the following circumstances.
- After antidepressant medication begins to raise the client's mood.
- After any sudden dramatic behavioral change (sudden cheerfulness, relief, freedom from guilt, or giving away personal belongings).
- Unstructured time on the unit. Times when the number of staff on the unit is limited.
- Reorient the client to person, place, and time as indicated (call the client by name, tell the client your name, tell the client where he or she is, and so forth).
- Spend time with the client.
- If the client is ruminating, tell him or her that you will talk about reality or about the client's feelings, but limit the attention given to repeated expressions of rumination.
- Initially, assign the same staff members to work with the client whenever possible.
- When approaching the client, use a moderate, level tone of voice.
- Avoid being overly cheerful.
- Use silence and active listening when interacting with the client.
- Let the client know that you are concerned and that you consider the client a worthwhile person.
- When first communicating with the client, use simple, direct sentences; avoid complex sentences or directions.
- Avoid asking the client many questions, especially questions that require only brief answers.
- Be comfortable sitting with the client in silence. Let the client know you are available to converse, but do not require the client to talk.
- Allow (and encourage) the client to cry. Stay with and support the client if he or she desires. Provide privacy if the client desires and it is safe to do so.
- Do not cut off interactions with cheerful remarks or platitudes (eg, "No one really wants to die," "Of course life is worth living," or "You'll feel better soon.").
- Do not belittle the client's feelings. Accept the client's verbalizations of feelings as real, and give support for this ventilation of feelings, especially for expressions of emotions that may be difficult for the client to accept in himself or herself (like anger).
- Encourage the client to ventilate feelings in whatever way is comfortable—verbal and nonverbal. Let the client know you will listen and accept what is being expressed.
- Interact with the client on topics with which he or she is comfortable.
- Do not probe for information.
- Teach the client about the problem solving process: explore possible options, examine the consequences of each alternative, select and implement an alternative, and evaluate the results.

- Provide positive feedback at each step of the process.
- If the client is not satisfied with the chosen alternative, assist the client to select another alternative.

Nursing Diagnosis	*Assessment Data*	*Expected Outcomes*
Impaired Social Interaction Insufficient or excessive quantity or ineffective quality of social exchange.	• Withdrawn behavior • Verbalization diminished in quantity, quality, or spontaneity • Rumination • Low self-esteem • Unsatisfactory or inadequate interpersonal relationships • Verbalizing or exhibiting discomfort around others • Social isolation • Inadequate social skills • Poor personal hygiene	• Communicate with others • Participate in activities

NURSING INTERVENTIONS

- Teach the client social skills, and encourage him or her to practice these skills with staff members and other clients.
- Give the client feedback regarding social interactions.
- Initially, interact with the client on a one-to-one basis.
- Progress to facilitating social interactions between the client and other clients, then in small groups and gradually larger groups.
- Encourage the client to pursue personal interests, hobbies, and recreational activities. Consultation with a recreational therapist may be indicated.
- Encourage the client to identify supportive people outside the hospital and to develop these relationships.

Nursing Diagnosis	*Assessment Data*	*Expected Outcomes*
Chronic Low Self-Esteem Longstanding negative self-evaluation/feelings about self or self-capabilities	• Feelings of inferiority • Defeatist thinking • Self-criticism • Lack of involvement • Minimizing of own strengths • Guilt Feelings of despair, worthlessness	• Verbalize increased feelings of self-worth • Express feelings directly and openly • Evaluate own strengths realistically

NURSING INTERVENTIONS

- Encourage the client to become involved with staff and other clients in the milieu through interactions and activities.
- Give the client positive feedback for completion of responsibilities, such as self-care activities and interactions with others.
- Involve the client in activities that are pleasant or recreational as a break from self-examination.
- If negativism dominates the client's conversations, it may be helpful to structure the content of the client's interactions.
- For example, make an agreement to listen to 10 minutes of "negative" interaction after which the client agrees to interact on more neutral or positive topics.
- At first, provide simple activities that can be accomplished easily and quickly.
- Begin with a project on the unit with the client alone; progress to group occupational and recreational therapy sessions.
- Give the client positive feedback for participation.
- Give the client honest praise for the accomplishment of small activities or individual responsibilities by realizing and acknowledging how difficult it can be for the client to perform these tasks.
- Gradually increase the number and complexity of activities or responsibilities expected of the client; give positive feedback at each level of accomplishment.
- It may be necessary to stress to the client that he or she should begin doing things to feel better, rather than waiting to feel better before doing things.
- Explore with the client his or her personal strengths.
- Making a written list is sometimes helpful.

4. OBSESSIVE-COMPULSIVE DISORDER

Nursing Diagnosis	*Assessment Data*	*Expected Outcomes*
Anxiety Vague uneasy feeling of discomfort or dread accompanied by an autonomic response (the source often nonspecific or unknown to the individual); a feeling of apprehension caused by anticipation of danger. It is an alerting signal that warns of impending danger and enables the individual to take measures to deal with the threat.	• Obsessive thoughts (may be destructive or delusional) • Compulsive, ritualistic behavior (eg, repeated hand-washing) • Self-mutilation or other physical problems (such as damage to skin from excessive washing) • Overemphasis on cleanliness and neatness • Fears • Guilt feelings • Denial of feelings	• Be free from self-inflicted harm • Demonstrate decreased anxiety, fears, guilt, rumination, or aggressive behavior

NURSING INTERVENTIONS

- The client may need to be secluded or restrained or otherwise protected when he or she attempts self-mutilation or harm.
- Try to substitute a physically safe behavior for harmful practices, even if the new behavior is compulsive or ritualistic. For example, if the client is cutting himself or herself, direct him or her toward tearing paper.
- If the client's behaviors are not harmful, try not to call attention to the compulsive acts initially.
- Encourage the client to verbally identify his or her concerns, life stresses, anxieties, fears, and so forth.
- Encourage the client to express his or her feelings in ways that are acceptable to the client (through talking, crying, physical activities, and so forth).
- If the client is ruminating (e.g., on his or her worthlessness), acknowledge the client's feelings, but then try to redirect the interaction in a positive direction.
- Discuss the client's specific perceptions of his or her feelings and possible ways to deal with these feelings.
- If the client continues to ruminate, withdraw your attention at that time (Tell the client that you will discuss other things, and state when you will return, or when you will be available for interaction again.)

5. ATTENTION-DEFICIT/HYPERACTIVITY DISORDER

Nursing Diagnosis	*Assessment Data*	*Expected Outcomes*
Risk for Injury At risk for injury as a result of environmental conditions interacting with the individual's adaptive and defensive resources	• Motorperceptual dysfunction, for example, poor hand eye coordination • Inability to perceive potentially harmful situations • Intrusive behavior with others • Impulsivity	Be free of injury or unnecessary risks Respond to limits regarding intrusion on others

NURSING INTERVENTIONS

- Talk with the client about safe and unsafe behavior.
- Explain to the client that accidents will result in increased supervision and that purposeful unsafe behavior will have consequences.
- Assess the frequency and severity of accidents.
- Provide supervision for potentially dangerous situations.

- Limit the client's participation in activities when safety cannot be ensured.
- Attempt to distinguish between accidents and behaviors that are deliberate.
- Assist the client's parents or care-givers to make the distinction between accidental and purposeful incidents.
- If the situation is determined to be accidental, institute safeguards or limitations as appropriate.
- If the situation is determined to be deliberate, institute consequences in a nonpunitive manner.
- Do not assume that the client knows proper or expected behavior.
- State expectations for behavior in clear terms.
- Make corrective feedback as specific as possible, for example, "Do not jump down the stairs. Walk down one step at a time."
- Provide consequences that are directly related to the undesirable behavior.
- Institute consequences as soon as possible after the occurrence of the behavior.

6. PHOBIAS

Nursing Diagnosis	*Assessment Data*	*Expected Outcomes*
Fear Response to perceived threat that is consciously recognized as a danger.	• Anticipatory anxiety (when thinking about the phobic object) • Panic anxiety (when confronted with the phobic object) • Avoidance behaviors that interfere with relationships or social or occupational functioning • Recognition of the phobia as irrational • Embarrassment over the phobic fear • Sufficient discomfort to seek treatment	• Verbalize feelings of fear and discomfort • Respond to relaxation techniques with decreased anxiety

NURSING INTERVENTIONS

- Allow the client to express feelings openly.
- Initially, it may be beneficial to focus on the client's feeling embarrassed, need to seek treatment, and so forth without discussing the phobic situation specifically.

- Teach the client and, family or significant others about phobic reactions.
- Dispel any myths that may be troubling the client. For example, it is common for others to tell the phobic individual that, all he or she has to do is face up to [the phobic situation] and he or she will get over it.
- Reassure the client that he or she can learn to decrease the anxiety and, gain control over the anxiety attacks.
- Reassure the client that he or she will not be forced to confront the phobic situation, until prepared to do so.
- Assist the client to distinguish between the phobic trigger and those problems related to avoidance behaviors that are interfering with daily life.
- Instruct the client progressive relaxation techniques. These include deep breathing, focusing on specific muscles to decrease tenseness, and imagining himself or herself in a quiet, peaceful place.
- Encourage the client to practice relaxation until he or she is comfortable and successful.
- Explain systematic desensitization thoroughly to the client .
- Reassure the client that, you will allow him or her as much time as needed at each step.
- Have the client develop a hierarchy of situations that, relate to the phobia.
- Have the client rank the list, in order from the least anxiety producing situation for the client (For example, a client with a phobia of dogs might rank situations beginning with looking at a picture of a dog, up to actually petting a dog.)
- Begin with the least anxiety-producing situation.
- Have the client use progressive relaxation in that situation until he or she is able to decrease the anxiety.
- When the client is comfortable with that situation, go to the next item on the list, and repeat the procedure.
- If the client becomes excessively anxious or begins to feel out of control, return to the former step with which the client was comfortable and successful, and proceed slowly to subsequent steps.
- Give positive feedback for the client's efforts at each step.
- Convey the idea that he or she is succeeding at each step.
- Avoid equating success only with mastery of the entire process.
- Discuss the previously identified avoidance behaviors with the client to determine, if there is a corresponding decrease, as the client progresses in systematic desensitization.
- It may be necessary to address specific avoidance behavior, if any persist after the client has completed the desensitizing process.

7. SUICIDAL BEHAVIOR

Nursing Diagnosis	*Assessment Data*	*Expected Outcomes*
Risk for Suicide • At risk for selfinflicted, lifethreatening injury.	• Suicidal ideas, feelings, ideation, plans, gestures, or attempts • Lack of impulse control • Lack of future orientation • Self-destructive tendencies • Feelings of anger or hostility • Agitation • Aggressive behavior • Feelings of worthlessness, hopelessness, or despair • Guilt • Anxiety • Sleep disturbance • Substance use • Perceived or observable loss • Social isolation • Problems of depression, withdrawn behavior, eating disorders, psychotic behavior, personality disorder, manipulative behavior, posttraumatic stress, or other psychiatric problems	• Not harm himself or herself or others • Identify alternative ways of dealing with stress and emotional problems

NURSING INTERVENTIONS

- Determine the appropriate level of suicide precautions for the client.
- Institute these precautions immediately on admission (may be by nursing order or by physician order). Some suggested levels of precautions follow:
  —The client has one-to-one contact with a staff member at all times, even when going to the bathroom and sleeping. The client is restricted to the unit and is permitted to use nothing that may cause harm to him or her (e.g., sharp objects, a belt).
  —Special attention—the client's whereabouts and activities on the unit should be known at all times. The client must be accompanied by a staff member while off the unit but may be in a staff-client group.

—Assess the client's suicidal potential, and evaluate the level of suicide precautions at least daily.
—In your initial assessment, note any previous suicide attempts and methods, as well as family history of mental illness or suicide. Obtain this information in a matter-of-fact manner; do not discuss at length or dwell on details.
—Ask the client if he or she has a plan for suicide.
—Attempt to ascertain how detailed and feasible the plan.
—Explain suicide precautions to the client.
—Be especially alert to sharp objects and other potentially dangerous items (eg, glass containers, ashtrays, vases, matches, and lit cigarettes); items like these should not be in the client's possession.

- The client's room should be centrally located, preferably near the nurses' station and within view of the staff.
- Avoid placing the client in a room at the end of a hallway or near an exit, elevator, or stairwell.
- Make sure that windows are locked so that the client cannot open them (in a general hospital the maintenance department may have to seal or otherwise secure the windows).
- If it is necessary for the client to use a sharp object, sign out the object to the client, and stay with the client during its use.
- Have the client use an electric shaver if possible.
- If the client is attempting to harm himself or herself, it may be necessary to restrain the client or to place him or her in seclusion with no objects that can be used to self-inflict injury (electric outlets, silverware, and even bed clothing).
- Know the whereabouts of the client at all times.
- Designate a specific staff person to be responsible for the client at all times.
- If this person must leave the unit for any reason, information and responsibility regarding supervision of the client must be transferred to another staff person.
- Stay with the client when he or she is meeting hygienic needs such as bathing, shaving, and cutting nails.
- Check the client at frequent, irregular intervals during the night to ascertain the client's safety and whereabouts.
- Maintain especially close supervision of the client at any time there is a decrease in the number of staff, the amount of structure, or the level of stimulation (nursing report at the change of shift, mealtime, weekends, nights).
- Also, be especially aware of the client during any period of turmoil or distraction and when clients are going to and from activities.
- Be alert to the possibility of the client saving up his or her own medications or obtaining medications or dangerous objects from other clients or from visitors.
- You may need to check the client's mouth after medication administration or use liquid medications to ensure that they are ingested.

- Observe, record, and report any changes in the client's mood (elation, withdrawal, sudden resignation).
- Observe the client, and note behavior patterns with regard to the time of day, structured versus unstructured time, interactions with others, tasks, activities, responsibilities, and attention span.
- Use this information to plan nursing care and the client's activities (e.g., observe when the client is more animated or withdrawn).
- Be aware of the relationships the client is forming with other clients; note who may become his or her confidant.
- Be alert to any manipulative or attention-seeking behavior
- *Note:* The client may ask you not to tell anyone something he or she tells you. Avoid promising to keep secrets in this way; make it clear to the client that you must share all information with the other staff members on the treatment team, but assure the client of confidentiality with regard to anyone outside the treatment team.
- Tell the client that although you are willing to discuss emotions or other topics, you will not discuss details of prior suicide attempts repeatedly; discourage such conversations with other clients also.
- Encourage the client to talk about his or her feelings, relationships, or life situation.
- Convey that you care about the client and that you believe the client is a worthwhile human being.
- Be alert to the client's behaviors, especially decreased communication, conversations about death or the futility of life, disorientation, low frustration tolerance, dependency and dissatisfaction with dependence, disinterest in surroundings, and concealing articles that could be used to harm self.
- Do not joke about death, belittle the client's wishes or feelings, or make insensitive remarks, such as "Everybody really wants to live."
- Do not belittle the client's prior suicide attempts, which other people may deem "only" attention-seeking gestures.
- Do not make moral judgments about suicide or reinforce the client's feelings of guilt or sin.
- Referral to the facility chaplain, clergy, or other spiritual resource person may be indicated.
- Examine and remain aware of your own feelings regarding suicide.
- Talk with other staff members to deal with these feelings if necessary.
- Involve the client as much as possible in planning his or her own treatment.
- Convey your interest in the client. Seek out the client for interaction at least once per shift.
- If the client says, "I don't feel like talking," "I don't want to talk to you," or "Leave me alone," remain with the client in silence or state that you will be back later to talk or be with the client, and then withdraw.
- You may tell the client that you will return at a specific time.

- Encourage and support the client's expression of anger. (*Remember:* Do not take the anger personally.)
- Help the client deal with the fear of expressing anger, the fear of subsequent consequences and feelings, and so forth.
- Support the client in expressing anger or making plans to directly express anger when it occurs.
- Examine with the client his or her home environment and relationships outside the hospital.
- that, if any, changes should occur to decrease the likelihood of future suicidal behavior? Include the client's family or significant others in teaching, skill development, and therapy, if indicated.
- Plan with the client how he or she will recognize and deal with feelings and situations that have precipitated suicidal feelings or behavior in the past. Include whom the client will contact (ideally, identify someone in the home environment), where to go, what things may alleviate suicidal feelings (identify what has worked in the past).

8. POST-TRAUMATIC STRESS DISORDER

Nursing Diagnosis	*Assessment Data*	*Expected Outcomes*
Post-Trauma Syndrome Sustained maladaptive response to a traumatic, overwhelming event	• Flashbacks or re-experiencing the traumatic event(s) • Nightmares or recurrent dreams of the event or other trauma • Sleep disturbances (e.g., insomnia, early awakening, crying out in sleep) • Depression • Denial of feelings or emotional numbness • Projection of feelings • Difficulty in expressing feelings • Anger (may not be overt) • Guilt or remorse • Low self-esteem • Frustration and irritability	• Identify the traumatic event • Demonstrate decreased physical symptoms • Verbalize need to grieve • Establish an adequate balance of rest, sleep, and activity • Demonstrate decreased anxiety, fear, guilt, and so forth Participate in treatment program

Contd...

Contd...

Nursing Diagnosis	*Assessment Data*	*Expected Outcomes*
	• Anxiety, panic, or separation anxiety • Fears—may be displaced or generalized (as in fear of men in rape victims) • Decreased concentration • Difficulty expressing love or empathy • Difficulty experiencing pleasure • Difficulty with interpersonal relationships, marital problems, divorce • Abuse in relationships • Sexual problems • Substance use • Employment problems • Physical symptoms	

NURSING INTERVENTIONS

- When you approach the client, be nonthreatening and professional.
- Initially, assign the same staff members to the client if possible; try to respect the client's feelings regarding gender issues at this time.
- Gradually increase the number and variety (including gender) of staff members interacting with the client.
- Educate yourself and other staff members about the client's experience and about post-traumatic behavior.
- Examine and remain aware of your own feelings regarding both the client's traumatic experience, and his or her feelings and behavior at the present time.
- Talk with other staff members to ventilate, and work through your feelings.
- Remain nonjudgmental in your interactions with the client.
- Be consistent with the client; convey acceptance of him, or her as a person while setting, and maintaining limits regarding behaviors.
- Assess the client's history of substance use (information from significant others might be helpful).
- Be aware of the client's use or abuse of substances while hospitalized.
- Determine and enforce consequences for this behavior; it may be helpful to allow the client or client group to have input into these decisions.

- If substance use is a major problem for the client, referral to a substance dependence treatment program may be appropriate.
- Encourage the client to talk about his or her experience(s); be accepting and nonjudgmental of the client's accounts and perceptions.
- Encourage the client to express his or her feelings through talking, writing, crying, or other ways in which the client is comfortable.
- Especially encourage the expression of anger, guilt, and rage.
- Teach the client and the family or significant others about posttraumatic behavior and treatment.
- As tolerated, encourage the client to share his or her feelings and experiences in group therapy, in a support group related to post-trauma, or with other clients informally.
- Give the client positive feedback for expressing feelings and sharing experiences. Remain nonjudgmental toward the client.
- If the client has a religious or spiritual orientation, referral to a member of the clergy, or a chaplain may be appropriate.
- Encourage the client to make realistic plans for life outside the hospital and to make appropriate changes integrating his or her traumatic experience.
- Provide education about and practice with stress reduction or stress management techniques, relaxation techniques, assertiveness training, self defense training (for rape survivors), and development of other skills as appropriate.
- Provide social skills and leisure time counseling, or refer the client to a recreational therapist as appropriate.
- Talk with the client about employment, including his or her history of employment, job-related stress, problems with authority figures, and so forth. Refer the client to vocational services as needed.
- Help the client arrange for follow-up therapy as needed. Referral to a therapist or groups that specialize in PTSD, rape or incest survival, sexual issues, and so forth may be indicated.

9. ALCOHOL

Nursing Diagnosis	*Assessment Data*	*Expected Outcomes*
Ineffective Health Maintenance Inability to identify, manage, and/or seek out help to maintain health.	• Physical symptoms (impaired nutrition, fluid and electrolyte imbalance, gastrointestinal disturbances, liver impairment) • Physical exhaustion • Sleep disturbances • Dependence on alcohol	• Establish nutritious eating patterns • Establish physiologic homeostasis • Establish a balance of rest, sleep, and activity Maintain personal hygiene and grooming

NURSING INTERVENTIONS

- Monitor the client's health status based on predetermined parameters or rating scale.
- Administer medications as ordered or as indicated by alcohol withdrawal protocol.
- Observe the client for any behavioral changes as well.
- Alert the physician to any changes observed or when assessments exceed established parameters.
- Complete the physical assessment of the client; ask what and how much the client usually drinks, as well as the time and amount of the last drink of alcohol.
- Offer fluids frequently, especially juices and malts.
- Serve only decaffeinated coffee.
- Intravenous therapy may be indicated for clients in severe withdrawal.
- Monitor the client's fluid and electrolyte balance.
- Provide food or nourishing fluids as soon as the client can tolerate eating; have something available at night (Bland food usually is tolerated more easily at first).
- Administer medication to minimize the progression of withdrawal or complications and to facilitate sleep.
- Encourage the client to bath, wash his or her hair, and wear clean clothes.
- Assist the client as necessary; it may be necessary to provide complete physical care, depending on the severity of the client's withdrawal.
- Teach the client that alcoholism is a disease that requires long-term treatment and follow-up.
- Refer the client to a substance dependence treatment program.
- Refer the client's family or significant others to Alanon, Alateen, or Adult Children of Alcoholics, as indicated.

Chapter 4

THEORIES

1. THEORIES OF PHYSICAL DEVELOPMENT-MATURATION OF THE CENTRAL NERVOUS SYSTEM: COMPARING LAUGUAGE, PERCEPTION, AND MOTOR SKILLS

Average Age	*Language Achievements*	*Perceptual Achievements*	*Motor Achievements*
Gestational		Can hear sounds	can swallow, suck thumb move limbs
Infancy Birth-3 months	Understands phenomes; responds to sound; can distinguish speech sounds Chomsky's language acquisition device Cooing; turn taking	Sound, touch, smell, taste present in newborns; sees patterns and shape, contrast	Balances head; lifts by arms
2 months	with caregivers	All perceptions more acute	Rolls side to side; reaches for object
16-28 weeks 28-40 weeks	Knows friendly from unfriendly voices Native language discrimination	Seeing more focused; sees all colors and patterns; vision and hearing coordinated Responds to motion; size constant; sees depth	Sits, pokes; crawls, plays pat-a-cake

Contd....

Contd....

Average Age	*Language Achievements*	*Perceptual Achievements*	*Motor Achievements*
6 months 40 weeks-year	Babbling; self-expressions for needs Words connected to meaning; first words. First sentence—two	Can see features Child sees at 20/100 at 6 months	Stands, walks, builds
1½-2½ years	words; 50 word vocabulary Three-word sentences;	Tracks objects	Scribbles,
Early childhood 2-3 years	uses small words, morphemes, to alter meaning; marked rise in vocabulary; girls greater	Intermodal developing between perceptions	Sphincter control; jumps; laterality appears.
3-5 years	Subtleties of tone and inflection; vocabulary increases to 14,000 words	Perceptual pathways integrated; Intermodal functions well developed	Tricycle, self-dependent, copies circles; fine motor developed, pencil, scissors
5 years	End of baby talk; end of second language ease Child can make self		Full postural control
Middle childhood 6-11 years	Metalinguistics understood; child improves inflection, pronouncement		Boys better gross motor skills; girls overall more developed
Adolescence 11 years and older			Gains in gross motor performance; girls' gross motor performance tapers at age 14; boys spurt through teens

2. THEORIES OF SOCIAL DEVELOPMENT AND SKILLS IN INFANTS AND CHILDREN

Approximate Ages	*Erik Erikson's Social Stages (Psychosexually Influenced)*	*Social Behaviors*
Infancy: 0-2 years 0-6 weeks 6 wecks-8 months		Infant recognizes caregiver's smell, voice Infant knows caregiver as different
5 months-1 year 8 months-2 years		Infant distingulshes self from caregiver Infant shows separation anxiety
18 months-2 years 0-1 year	Basic trust vs. mistrust	Child reapproaches parent, object constancy Infant develops trust based upon caretakers' attitudes and ability to provide
Early childhood: 2-5 years 2 years on		Child separates when given clear goals
1-3 years	Autonomy vs. shame	Child develops autonomy when allowed to do things without coercion and without undue help from caregivers
Middle childhood: 3-6 years 4-9 Years		Child assumes friends feels same as self Child's sense of purpose develops Child makes comparisons in terms of self-esteem Child understands different views Can understand when a friend likes a different game
6-11 Years 7-12 Years	Industry vs. inferiority	Competency develops through success at home and at school; parents not sole authority Drop in self-esteem with social referencing Can understand other person's viewpoint

Contd....

Contd....

Approximate Ages	*Erik Erikson's Social Stages (Psychosexually Influenced)*	*Social Behaviors*
Adolescence: 11-19 years 10-15 Years 12-19 Years 14 Year on	Identify vs. identity diffusion	Can get motivations; can use nonparents as role models Point of view for third party Can understand group of peers Secure personal identity; wants independence Knows values and personal goals Person sees that systems affect people Can see issues through social value context

3. THEORIES AND SKILLS OF COGNITIVE DEVELOPMENT IN INFANTS AND CHILDREN

Period of Development	*Plaget's Cognnitive Spatial Stages*	*Cognitive Achievements*
Gestational		Fetus can "learn" sounds and respond differentially to them after birth
Infancy: birth-2 years	Sensorimotor Includes concepts: Reflective; egocentric (newer research refutes this)	Infants "think" with their eyes, ears, senses Newborns can learn to associate stroking with sucking
Birth—1 month 1-4 months	Primary circular: Imitation, smiles, playful	Newborns can learn to suck to produce certain visual displays or music
4-8 months	Secondary circular: looks for objects partially hidden	Can remember for 1-month periods Can play with parent by looking for partially hidden objects
8-12 months	Secondary circulation coordinated: peek-a-boo, finds hidden objects	Memory Improves Body parts used as objects Can stack one object within another Remembers hidden objects

Contd....

Contd....

Period of Development	*Plaget's Cognnitive Spatial Stages*	*Cognitive Achievements*
12-18 months	Tertiary circular: explores properties and drops objects	Drops objects over crib Knows animal sounds; names objects
18 months-2 years	Mental representation, make-believe play; memory of objects	Knows body parts and familiar pictures Can understand causes not visible
Early childhood: 2-5 years 2-7 years	Preoperational Includes concepts: Egocentrism: "Iwant you to eat this too" Animistic: I'm afraid of the moon" Lack hierarchy: "Where do these blocks go" Centration: "I want it now, not after dinner" Irreversibility: "I don't know how to go back to that room"	Preschoolers use symbols Development of language and make believe No sign of logic 3-year-olds can count 2 to 3 objects; know colors and age4-year-olds can fantasize without concrete props
2-5 years	Transductive reasoning: "We have to go this way because that's the way Daddy goes"	5-6-year-olds get humor; understand good and bad; can do some chores
Middle childhood: 6-11 years 6 yars onward		7-11-year-olds have good memory; recall; can solve problems
7-11 years	Concrete-operationalIncludes concepts: Hierarchical classification—arranges cars by types Reversibility—can play games backward and forward, checkers triple kings Conservation—lose two dimes can look (or same)	Children begin to think logically Understand conservation of matter Frozen milk same amount as melted Can organize objects intro hierarchies Children seem rational and organized

Contd....

Contd....

Period of Development	*Plaget's Cognnitive Spatial Stages*	*Cognitive Achievements*
Adolescence: 11-19 years 11 years onward	Decentration—worry about small details, obsessive Spatial operations—likes models for directionsHorizontal decalage—conservation of weight, logic Transitive inference—syllogisms; compare everything, brand names important Formal operationalIncludes concepts: Hypothetic-deductive reasoning; adolescent quick thinking or excuses Imaginary audience—everyone is looking at them Personal fable—Inflated opinion of themselves Prepositional thinking—logic	Abstraction and reason Can think of all possibilities

4. PSYCHOSEXUAL DEVELOPMENT: THEORIES OF PSYCHOSEXUAL DEVELOPMENT AND PSYCHOSEXUAL SKILLS

Periods of Growth	*Freudian Psychosexual Stages*	*Gender Identity*	*Gender Role*	*Gender Relationships*	*Psychosexual Skills*
Gestational-infancy: 0-2 years 0-1 year 1-1 years 1-2 years	Oral stage	Gender labeling	Stereotyping appears		Ego directs sucking needs Children label stereotypes: "Girls like dolls" Child can label self

Contd....

Contd....

Periods of Growth	*Freudian Psycho-sexual Stages*	*Gender Identity*	*Gender Role*	*Gender Relationships*	*Psychosexual Skills*
					picture, or other children's sex using clothes, toys, hair, activities
Early childhood: 2-5 years					Child enjoys control over bowels
1-3 years	Anal stage.	Gender stability		Sex not issue- with peer choice Sex "play" common	Child knows that gender label stays as part of self but does not see it as constant "I'm not doing that. Don't make me a girl" child sees activities related to gender not causing gender
3 years					
5 years		Gender fixed usually	Stereotyping fixed at age 5 but becomes less rigid with growth		
Middle childhood: 5-11 years 3-6 years	Phallic stage	Gender consistency		Same-sex peers favored Same-sexplay- "doctor"	Child's id transferred to genitalsChild now knows gender remains "I'm going to wear that hat, even if it is a boys" Issues with Oedipus and Electra
6-11 years	Latency stage	Gender constancy	Child focuses on social cues to recognize gender	Increased masturbation Increased heterosexual play	Superego consolidates conscienceGender remains constant regardless of clothing or behavior
Adolescence: 11-19 years 12-19 years	Genital stage			Sexual activity begins	Sexual activity increases

5. EMOTIONAL DEVELOPMENT THEORIES OF EMOTIONAL DEVELOPMENT AND EMOTIONAL SKILLS

Stages First Seen	*(Integrated Theory) Acquisition of Basic Emotions*	*(Adaptive Theory) Anna Freud's Model Defenses As Tools for Emotional Growth*	*Emotional Behavior*
Gestational-Infacy; 0-2 years 0-2 months on 3-4 months on 7-12 months 1-2 years	 Stage 1: Innatge emotions, emotional responsiveness Stage 2: Self-conscious emotional reactivity	 Displacement, suppression	• Social smile and joy shown Responds to emotions of others • All emotions there • Laughter possible and more control over smiles; anger shown • Able to elicit more responsiveness • Denies to cope with stress. • Some indications of empathy starting expressions of feeling, "I like you, Daddy" "I'm sorry" • Likes attention and approval; enjoys play alone or next to peers
Early childhood: 2-5 years 3-6 years	 Stage 3: Emotional self-awareness connecting emotion with effects	 Identification, projection. Repression	• Empathy increases with understanding • More response and less reaction; self-regulation, "Use your words to say that you are angry with him" • Aggression becomes competition By age 5 shows sensitivity to criticism and *care* about feelings of others
Middle childhood: 5-11 years 7-11 years	 Stage 4: Emotional responsiveness to feelings of others		• Ego rules until age 6 • Empathy becomes altruism, "I feel so bad about their fire, I'm going to give them some of my things" • Super ego dominates

6. MORAL DEVELOPMENT—KOHLBERG

Moral development is influenced by a child's motivation or need, the child's opportunity to learn social roles, and from the forms of justice the child encounters in the social institutions where he or she lives.

Level	*Age (Year)*	*Stage*	*Development Issues*
I. Preconventional (selfcentered Orientation)	4-10	1. Punishment obedience orientation 2. Hedonistic and instrumental orientation	• Moral decisions based on avoidance of punishment • Moral decisions motivated by desire for rewards rather than avoiding punishment, and belief that by helping others they will get help in return
II. Conventional (able to see victim's perspective)	10-13 but can to into adoles-cence	3. Good boy/ girl orientation 4. Law and order orientation	• Moral decisions based on desire for approval from others Moral decisions based on desire for approval from others thing • Moral decisions defined by rights, assigned duty, rules of community, and respect for authority
III. Postconventional (underlying ethical principles are considered that take into account societal needs)		5. Social contract orientation 6. Hierarchy of principles orientation	• Moral decisions based on a sense of community respect and disrespect. Rules should be followed to maintain community harmony. • Moral judgments are based on principles of justice, the reciprocity and quality of human rights, and respect for dignity of human beings as individual persons: Golden rule—do to others as you would have them do to you.

Chapter 5

CASE RECORD FORMAT

PSYCHOSIS CASE RECORD

1. Name: ....
2. Father's/Husband's Name: ....
3. Address...
4. Distance from the health centre...
5. Age: yr 6. Sex: Male/Female 7. Date of registration ....
8. Mode of referral:
   - i. Health worker-Name : ....
   - ii. Other patient:
   - iii. Self:
   - iv. Identified in the clinic:
   - v. Others (specify)...
9. Duration of illness: (Encircle the appropriate number)
   - i. Less than 1 week
   - ii. 1 week - 1 month
   - iii. 1 - 3 months
   - iv. 3 - 6 months
   - v. 6 months - 1 year
   - vi. 1 - 3 years
   - vii. 3-5 years
   - viii. More than 5 years
   - ix. Not known
10. Mode of onset
    - i. Sudden
    - ii. Gradual
    - iii. Not known
11. Precipitating factor: i. Present ii. Absent

    If present, details...
12. Associated events
    - i. Fever
    - ii. Alcohol/Drug intake
    - iii. Head injury
    - iv. Physical illness
13. Type of illness:
    - i. Continuous
    - ii. Episodic
14. Symptoms: (Encircle the symptom which is present)
    - i. Excessive activity
    - ii. Violence
    - xiii. Fear/anxiety
    - xiv. Lack of interest

iii.	Bizarre behaviors	xv.	Anger/irritability
iv.	Dull/withdrawn	xvi.	No emotion
v.	Too much speech	xvii.	Suicidal ideation
vi.	Too little speech	xviii.	Suicidal attempt
vii.	Irrelevant speech	xix.	Disorientation
viii.	Ununderstandable speeches	xx.	Loss of memory
ix.	Firm, false belief	xxi.	Sleep of disturbance
x.	Suspicion	xxii.	Lack of memory
xi.	Elation/excess happiness	xxiii.	Self neglect
xii.	Sadness	xxiv.	Sexual problems

xxv. Somatic pains (Mention)..

xxvi. Any other: (Specify)...

15. Past history of mental illness — i. Present — ii. Absent
    If present, type — i. Psychosis — ii. Neurosis
16. Family history of psychosis — i. Present — ii. Absent
17. Signs

a.	Sensorium	i. Clear	ii. Clouded	iii. Unconscious
b.	Appearance	i. Clean	ii. Unclean	
c.	Behaviour	i. Restless iv. Normal	ii. Dull	iii. Suspicious
d.	Talk	i. Normal iv. Irrelevant	ii. Too much	iii. Too less
e.	Delusion	i. Present	ii. Absent	
f.	Hallucination	ii. Present	ii. Absent	
g.	Mood	i. Elated iv. No emotion	ii. Sad v. Normal	iii. Angry
h.	Suicidal	i. Severe iv. Nil	ii. Moderate	iii. Mild
i.	Memory disturbance	i. Present	ii. Absent	
j.	Insight	i. Present	ii. Absent	iii. Partial
k.	Physical exam (specify)	i. Normal	ii. Abnormal	

l. Any other, specify...

18. Diagnosis i. Schizophrenia — ii. Mania — iii. Depression
    iv. Organic psychosis — v. Other psychosis
19. Mode of management: i. Managed at PHC
    ii. Refer to a bigger hospital
20. Treatment: i. Drugs — ii. Drugs + Counseling
    iii. Counseling only

21. Drugs prescribed:

....

....

Health Center: Signature of the MOH

NEUROSIS CASE RECORD

1. Name:..
2. Father's/Husband's Name:..
3. Address ....
4. Distance from the health centre..
5. Age:..........yr 6. Sex : Male/Female 7. Date of registration :...........................
8. Mode of referral:
   - i. Health worker-Name : ....
   - ii. Other patient
   - iii. Self
   - iv. Identified in the clinic
   - v. Others (specify)...
9. Duration of symptoms :
   - i. Less than 1 week
   - ii. 1 week - 1 month
   - iii. 1 - 3 months
   - iv. 3 - 6 months
   - v. 6 months - 1 year
   - vi. 1 - 3 years
   - vii. 3 - 5 years
   - viii. More than 5 years
   - ix. Not known
10. Mode of onset i. Sudden ii. Gradual iii. Not known
11. Precipitating factor: i. Present ii. Absent

    If present, details..
12. Symptoms : (Tick whichever present)
   - i. Fear
   - ii. Palpitation
   - iii. Giddiness
   - xii. Suicidal attempt
   - xiii. Fits/Falling unconscious
   - xiv. Other History symptoms (specify)....................

iv. Increased sweating
v. Dryness of mouth
vi. Tremors
vii. Difficulty to concentrate
viii. Impaired memory
ix. Sadness
x. Lack of interest
xi. Death wish/suicidal ideation
xv. Headache
xvi. Other body aches/pains
xvii. Weakness
xviii. Fatigability
xix. No/less appetite
xx. Sleep disturbance
xxi. Sexual problems (specify)............
xxii. Others (specify) ....

13. Stress factors:
    i. Family
    ii. Financial
    iii. Occupation
    iv. Sexual
    v. Others (specify)..
    vi. Absent...
    Details...
14. On examination:
    i. Signs of anxiety
    ii. Signs of depression
    iii. Physical illness (specify)...
    iv. Normal
15. Insight:
    i. Present
    ii. Absent
    iii. Partial
16. Diagnosis :
    i. Anxiety neurosis
    ii. Depressive neurosis
    iii. Hysteria
    iv. Others (specify)...........................
17. Treatment:
    i. Drugs
    ii. Drugs & Counseling
    iii. Counseling
18. Drugs prescribed :

....

....

19. Psychological help :

....

Health Center: Signature of the MOH

MENTAL RETARDATION CASE RECORD

1. Name: ....
2. Age:..................................yr 3. Sex: Male/Female
4. Father's Name: ....
5. Address ....
6. Distance from the health centre..
7. Mode of referral:
   i. Health worker-Name:..
   ii. Other patient iii. Self/family iv. Others
8. Date of registration :
   i. Poor motor development ii. Delayed milestones
   iii. Dull iv. Hyperactive
   v. Speech problems vi. Physical handicaps
   vii. Fits viii. Scholastic backwardness
9. Lack of self care
   i. Lack of social sense
   ii. Other (specify) ....
10. Present:
    i. Since birth
    ii. Later in life (specify the age of onset)...
11. Consanguinity among the parents : i. Present ii. Absent
    iii. Not known
12. Family history of: i. Mental illness ii. Mental retardation
    iii. Epilepsy iv. Nil
13. Mother's health :
    a. Age at pregnancy (for this child):
       i. Below 30 years % ii. 31-40 yrs. iii. 41 years +
    b. Birth order:
       i. First ii. Second iii. Third
       iv. Fourth v. Fifth vi. Sixth and above (specify)...........
    c. Prenatal: i. Healthy ii. Poor nutrition
       iii. Illness (specify)
    d. Natal:
       i. Difficult labour
       ii. Forceps/caesarian iii. Delayed birth cry
       iv. Signs of hypoxia v. Premature.
    e. Postnatal (child)
       i. Poor nutrition ii. Fits
       iii. Infection iv. Head injury

14. Developmental milestones: Delayed Normal
    - i. Holding neck erect:
    - ii. Sitting :
    - iii. Standing :
    - iv. Walking :
    - v. Speech :
15. Physical examination : i. Normal ii. Abnormal (details)

....

....

....

16. Abilities of the child : (Tick the appropriate)
    - i. Able to stand
    - ii. Able to walk
    - iii. Toilet control
    - iv. Able to feed itself
    - v. Able to dress itself
    - vi. Able to speak
    - vii. Able to do simple work
    - viii. Others (specify)..............................
17. Diagnosis:
    - i. Mild M.R.
    - ii. Moderate M.R
    - iii. Severe M.R.
18. Associate problems :
    - i. Behavioral problems
    - ii. Hyperactivity
    - iii. Physical handicap
    - iv. Epilepsy
19. Treatment:
    - i. Drugs (specify)...
    - ii. Counseling ....
    - iii. Immediate task of training advised (specify)

....

....

Health Center: Signature of the MOH

EPILEPSY CASE RECORD

1. Name :..

2. Age...yr

3. Sex: Male/Female.............................

4. Father's/Husband's Name :...

5. Address : ....

6. Distance from health centre ....

7. Date of registration :

8. Mode of referral:

   i. Health worker-Name :..

   ii. Other patient

   iii. Self

   iv. Identified in the clinic

   v. Others

9. Duration of illness

   i. less than 1 week

   ii. 1 week/month

   iii. 1 - 3 months

   iv. 3 - 6 months

   v. 6 months - 1 year

   vi. 1 - 3 years

   vii. Up to 5 years

   viii. More than 5 years

   ix. Not known

10. Frequency of fits:

per day per month per year

11. Cluster/status: i. Present ii. Absent

12. Last attack on: ....

13. Description of the attack.- Put a tick mark against the relevant items:
    i. Aura
    ii. Focal onset
    iii. Unconsciousness
    iv. Sudden fall
    v. Injuries
    vi. Tonic /clonic movements (regular, synchronous)
    vii. Tongue bite-bleeding
    viii. Urinary /foecal incontinence
    ix. Post ictal symptoms
    x. Attack during sleep when alone
    xi. At specific time/places only
    xii. Changing pattern

14. Associated events: i. Fever ii. Hot water bath
    iii. Head injury iv. Alcohol intake v. Physical illness ....

15. On examination:

    i. An attack precipitated by sussetion

    ii. Neurological deficits present

    iii. Normal

16. Past history of epilepsy:
    i. Present ii. Absent

17. Family history of epilepsy:
    i. Present ii. Absent

18. Diagnosis:

i. Major epilepsy
ii. Focal epilepsy
iii. Focal - Generalized
iv. T.L.E.
v. Febrile fits
vi. Others ....

19. Associated disorder:

i. M.R.
ii. Behavioral problems
iii. Neurosis
iv. Psychosis
v. Others..
vi. None.

20. Drugs :

i. Prescribed
ii. Not prescribed

21. Drugs prescribed :

Health Center:

Signature of MOH

FOLLOW-UP RECORD

1. Name : ....
2. Village : ....
3. Age : .... Years
4. Sex : Male/Female
5. Drugs prescribed : ....
....
....
....

Date	*Drug intake*	*Follow up detail*	*Drugs dispensed*	*Due on*

Chapter 6

CASE WORK

CHILD GUIDANCE CLINIC

INTRODUCTION

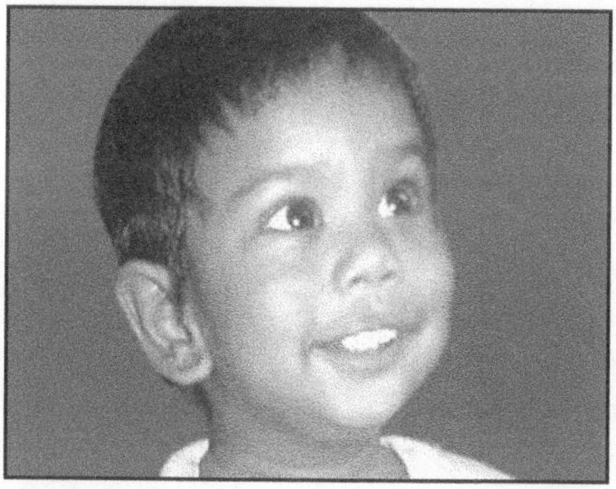

The mind's functions such as, Thinking, Feeling, Learning, Speaking, and Writing, are carried out by specific biochemicals in designated areas of the brain. Any developmental delay or later disregulation in these areas can cause Learning Disorders or Disabilities, Dyslexia, Attention Deficit, Hyperactivity Disorder (ADD/ADHD), Autism, Speech, and Language Disorders, etc., in children, as well as Behavior and Emotional Disorders.

GOALS

Children tend to have an **overlap** of Developmental, Neurological, Academic and Emotional disorders at the same time, in the same child. Therefore, a Team of Specialists from all related fields is required to evaluate children with difficulties.

TEAM

A **multi-disciplinary approach** is made possible in our **Child Guidance Clinic (CGC)** by having Clinical and Educational Psychologists, Social Workers, Special Educators, Language Pathologist, Speech Therapist, Neurologist, and Consultant Psychiatrists in the team for appropriate guidance or treatment.

THE SETTING

Child Guidance Clinic (CGC) works in the open setting that encourages Children and their Parents to walk in and seek help for Learning, and Behavior problems, Emotional problems, or Poor School Performance (PSP) without fear or stigma.

Services Include Professional Evaluation

- Poor School Performance (PSP) and Learning Disorders (LD)
- Levels of Intelligence (IQ) and Types of Intelligence
- Special Skills and Abilities
- Academic Skill Deficits in Reading, Writing, Spelling, Math, etc.
- Speech and Language Disorders: Stuttering, Aphasias, etc.
- Motor Skill Deficits; poor handwriting, clumsiness, etc.
- Attention Deficit Hyperactivity Disorders (ADD/ADHD)
- Defiant/Oppositional Behavior, Conduct Disorders
- Addiction to TV/Internet, Disorganized routines
- Tics/Tourette Disorder, 'Silent' Epilepsy
- Obsessive Behavior/Disorders; obsessive slowness/procrastination
- Anxiety, School Phobia, Exam Phobia and various Fears in the child
- Depression, Social Withdrawal, loss of interest
- Developmental Neurological Disorders
- 'Functional' symptoms like Headache, Breathlessness, Stomachache, Frequent sickness, Absenteeism from school, etc.

Stages of Evaluation: Protocol

1. Intake Interview.
2. Physical/Neurological Examination.
3. Assessment of Poor School Performance.
4. Assessing Overlapping Disorders.
5. Multidisciplinary Diagnosis and Documentation.

COMMUNITY PSYCHIATRY

DEFINITIONS

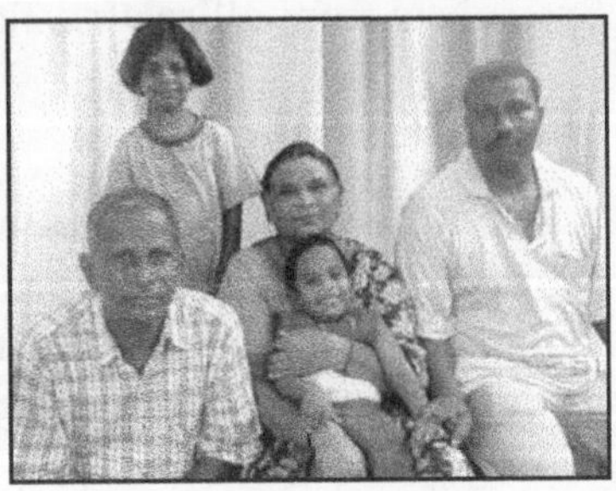

Community psychiatric nursing is the application of specialized knowledge, to populations and communities, to promote and maintain mental health, and to rehabilitate populations at risk that to have residual effects of mental illness.

The basic model of community mental health was defined by "General Caplan" in 1967.

GOALS

1. To provide prevention activities to population for promoting mental health.
2. To provide interventions as early as possible.

3. To develop innovative approaches to primary prevention activities.
4. To assit, in providing mental health education to populations, about mental health and illness.

Characteristics

1. Responsibility to a population for mental health care delivery
2. Treatment close to the patient in community based centers
3. Provision of comprehensive service
4. Multi-disciplinary team approaches
5. Providing continuity of care
6. Emphasis on prevention as well as treatment
7. Avoidance of unnecessary hospitalization.

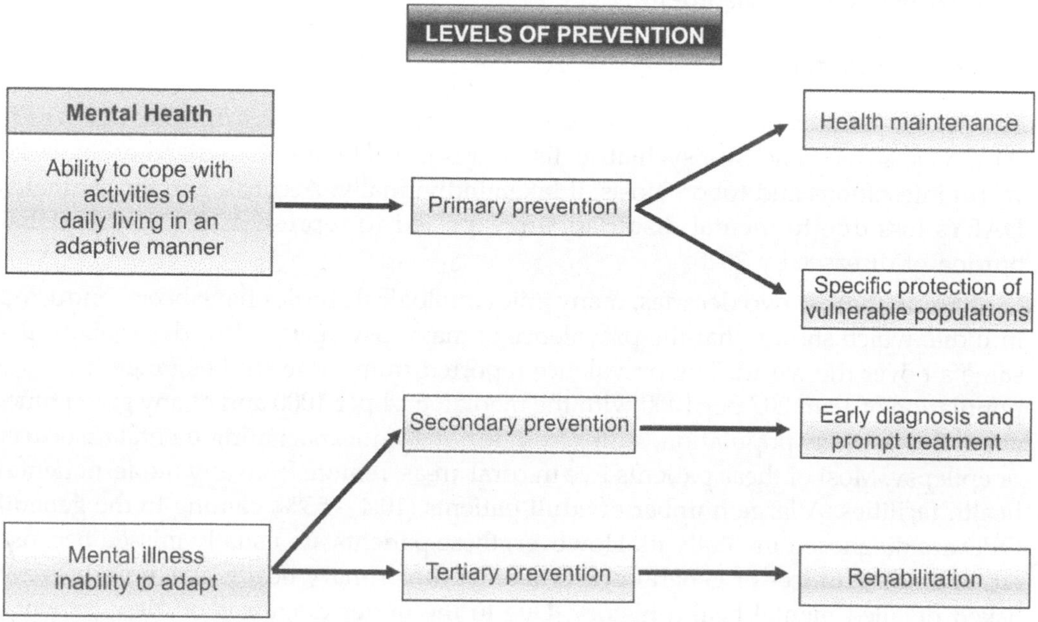

Role of nurse

1. Consultative role
2. Clinician role
3. Therapeutic role
4. Researcher role
5. Educator

6. Trainer/ manpower facilitators
7. Manager/Administrator
8. Domiciliary care
9. Liasons role
10. Preventive roles.

NATIONAL MENTAL HEALTH PROGRAMME

INTRODUCTION

Psychiatric symptoms are common in general population in both sides of the globe. These symptoms – worry, tiredness, and sleepless nights affect more than half of the adults at some time, while as many as one person in seven experiences some form of diagnosable neurotic disorder.

Burden of Disease

The World Bank report (1993), revealed that the "Disability Adjusted Life Year" (DALY) loss due to neuro-psychiatric disorder is much higher than diarrhea, malaria, worm infestations and tuberculosis, if taken individually. According to the estimates DALYs loss due to mental disorders are expected to represent 15% of the global burden of diseases by 2020.

During the last two decades, many epidemiological studies have been conducted in India, which shows, that the prevalence of major psychiatric disorder is about the same all over the world. The prevalence reported from these studies range from the population of 18 to 207 per 1000 with the median 65.4 per 1000 and at any given time, about 2–3 % of the population, suffer from seriously, incapacitating mental disorders or epilepsy. Most of these patients live in rural areas, remote from any modern mental health facilities. A large number of adult patients (10.4 – 53%) coming to the general OPD are diagnosed mentally ill. However, these patients are usually missed because either medical officer or general practitioner at the primary health care unit does not asked detailed mental health history. Due to the under diagnosis of these patients, unnecessary investigations and treatments are offered which heavily cost to the health providers.

Programme

The Government of India has launched the "National Mental Health Programme" (NMHP) in 1982, keeping in view the heavy burden of mental illness in the community, and the absolute inadequacy of mental health care infrastructure, in the country to deal with it.

Aims

1. Prevention and treatment of mental and neurological disorders and their associated disabilities.
2. Use of mental health technology to improve general health services.
3. Application of mental health principles in total national development to improve quality of life.

Objectives

1. To ensure availability and accessibility of minimum mental health care for all in the for seeable future, particularly to the most vulnerable and underprivileged sections of population.
2. To encourage application of mental health knowledge in general health care and in social development.
3. To promote community participation in the mental health services development, and to stimulate efforts towards self-help in the community.

Strategies

1. Integration mental health with primary health care through the NMHP;
2. Provision of tertiary care institutions for treatment of mental disorders;
3. Eradicating stigmatization of mentally ill patients and protecting their rights through regulatory institutions, like the "Central Mental Health Authority", and 'State Mental Health Authority'.

MENTAL HEALTH CARE

1. The mental morbidity requires priority in mental health treatment.
2. Primary health care at village and sub center level.
3. At Primary Health Center level.
4. At the District Hospital level.
5. Mental Hospital and Teaching Psychiatric Units.

District Mental Health Programme Components

1. Training programmes of all workers in the mental health team at the identified Nodal Institute in the State.
2. Public education in the mental health to increase, awareness and reduce stigma.
3. For early detection and treatment, the OPD and indoor services are provided.
4. Providing valuable data and experience at the level of community to the state and Centre for future planning, improvement in service and research.

Agencies like World Bank and WHO have been contacted to support various components of the programme. Funds are provided by the Govt. of India to the state governments and the nodal institutes to meet the expenditure on staff, equipments, vehicles, medicine, stationary, contingencies, training, etc. for initial 5 years and there after they should manage themselves. Govt. of India has constituted central 'Mental Health Authority' to oversee the implementation of the Mental Health Act 1986. It provides for creation of state 'Mental Health Authority' also to carry out the said functions.

The National Human Rights Commission also monitors the conditions in the mental hospitals along with the government of India and the states are currently acting on the recommendation of the joint studies conducted to ensure quality in delivery of mental care.

THRUST AREAS FOR 10TH FIVE-YEAR PLAN

1. District mental health programme in an enlarged and more effective form covering the entire country.
2. Streamlining/ modernization of mental hospitals in order to modify their present custodial role.
3. Upgrading department of psychiatry in medical colleges and enhancing the psychiatry content of the medical curriculum at the undergraduate as well as postgraduate level.
4. Strengthening the 'Central' and 'State Mental Health Authorities' with a permanent secretariat. Appointment of medical officers at state headquarters in order to make their monitoring role more effective.
5. Research and training in the field of community mental health, substance abuse and child/adolescent psychiatric clinics.

COMMENTS

1. For the first time in the last 40 years mental health has been chosen as the theme for the World Health Day 2001: "Mental Health: Stop Exclusion – Date to Care", Why? The recent evidence for the importance of mental health has been so striking that the WHO decided to give it, a priority during year 2001, the beginning of 21st century.
2. There is no initiative from the mental health professional to take active part in this programme. Most of them are not aware of the programme.
3. There is shortage of professional manpower and training programmes are not able to meet the demand in providing all medical private practitioners and medical officers.
4. Appropriate mental health can be provided at the subcentre and village level by minimum training of the health workers that will help in providing comprehensive health care at the most peripheral level.

5. The targets set for the programme are not achieved till today, after lapse of more than one decade. This indicates that there is a poor commitment of the government, psychiatrists, and community at large.
6. The programme has given more emphasis on the curative services to the mental disorders and preventive measures are largely ignored. More public awareness programmes are required.
7. The medical care in the hospitals are custodial in nature and this needs to be changed to a therapeutic approach.

Chapter 7

PREPARATION FOR ASSISTING WITH THERAPIES

ELECTROCOVULSIVE THERAPY (ECT)

DEFINITION

Electroconvulsive therapy is a type of, Somatic treatment first introduced, by Bini and Cerletti in April 1938. It is the artificial induction of a grandmal seizure through the application of electrical current, to the brain. The stimulus is applied through electrodes, that are placed either bilaterally in the fronto-temporal region, or unilaterally in the fronto-temporal region, or unilaterally on the non-dominant side.

MECHANISM OF ACTION

Exact mechanism is unknown.

- Produces biochemical change in brain.
- In level of norepinephrine and serotonin

ECT DEVICE

The apparatus used to convert, Ac main supply into stimulus, uses a step-down transformers to yield a choice of voltage ranging from 70 V to 180 V in steps of 10 volts. The stimulus during can be chosen from 0.1 sec to 1.0 sec in steps of 0.1 sec each or longer.

INDICATIONS

Psychotic depression, mania, catatonia, schizophrenia, severe depression, hyperactive mania, individuals who are extremely suicidal, etc.

CONTRAINDICATIONS

- Increased intracranial pressure
- Cerebral aneurysm/H/o cerebral hemorrhage
- H/o cardiovascular disease brain tumor.

- Acute myocardial infarction
- Congestive heart failure
- Pneumonia/aortic aneurysm.

ADMINISTRATION

- Hospital and clinic/nursing home.

ECT TEAM

- Psychiatrist, anesthesiologist, trained nurses and aides.

TREATMENT FACILITIES IN ECT ROOM

- ECT machine
- Anesthetic appliance
- Suction apparatus
- Face masks
- Oxygen cylinders with adjustable flow valves, curved tongue depressors, mouth gags
- Resuscitation apparatus
- Emergency drugs
- Defibrillator.

CONSENT

- Patient and legal guardian.

PRE-ECT PREPARATION

- Check the record for recent physical examination and routine lab investigation.
- Signed consent form.
- Information to family member and their involvement in the treatment.
- Communicate positive feeling to family.
- Discourage cigarette smoking—pulmonary secretion.
- Nil per oral—6 hr before treatment.
- Remove dentures, glasses, jawing, contact lens, metal hair clips, and pins.
- Dress—loose clothing.
- Empty bowel and bladder.
- Monitor vital signs.
- Administer atropine as ordered.
- Make sure that oxygen suction and ECT tube is available in case of emergency.
- Display warm and support to apprehension.

CARE DURING TREATMENT

Application of electrodes – Moistened with electrolyte gelley
- Interelectrode area
- Firm application of electrode
- Apply dry hands
- No contact with metallic parts of electrodes.

Electrode placement

1. Bilateral ECT – Each side 1 inch above the midpoint of an Imaginary line – outer canthus of eye and tragus.
2. In unilateral ECT, one electrode is placed on non dominant side, one inch lateral to vertex are used in unilateral and ECT.
3. Airway- mouth gag is inserted; neck is extended jaw pulled forward.
4. Usually 70 v to 150 v stimulus current is passed for a period of 0.1 to 0.5 sec.
5. Monitoring seizure activity – EEG monitoring - 'Cuff' method.
   - Re-oxygenating.
   - Maintaining airway and suctioning frequently.
   - Observe continuously and stay with the patient till he/she is fully awake.

CARE AFTER TREATMENT

- Side lying position with side rails.
- Touch and establish your presence when pt awakes up.
- Orient pt.
- Give medications for minor discomforts.
- Listen to patient's complaints.
- Promote normal activity.
- Provide food.
- Documentation of patient's responses.
- Check vital signs and record every fifteen minutes for the first hour.
- Ambulation.

SIDE EFFECTS

- Amnesia
- Confusion
- EEG
- Slowing
- Dizziness
- Dryness of mouth

- Headache
- Weakness/fatigue
- Muscle pain
- Nausea vomiting
- Palpitation
- Unsteady gait
- Poor concentration
- Drowsiness
- Anxiety
- Restlessness
- Sweating
- Respiratory distress
- Seizures
- Tongue bite
- Incontinence.

COMPLICATIONS

- Back pain, fractures, cardiac dysarhythmia in patient's with H/o coronary disease, respiratory distress, memory loss.

PSYCHOMETRIC ASSESSMENT

INTRODUCTION

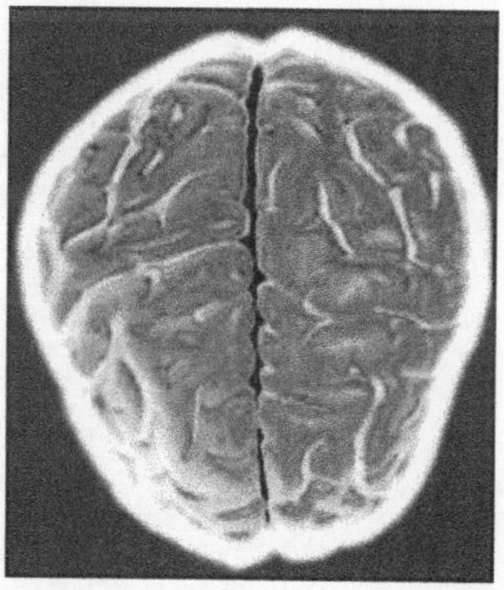

Psychometric and neurological tests are designed to measure specific aspects of people's intelligence, thinking, or personality.

Intelligence testing is necessary to establish the degree of mental retardation.

Neuro psychological tests help to quantify and localize brain damage.

Psychometric tests are used in the workplace to assist in the prediction of behaviors and performance. They are used in recruitment, selection, development, coaching, career counseling, and team-building.

TYPES OF TEST

1. Achievement and aptitude tests.
2. Intelligence test.
3. Neuro psychological test.

4. Occupational test.
5. Personality test.
6. Specific clinical test.

APTITUDE TEST

1. **Achievement and aptitude tests** are usually in education or employment setting, and they attempt to measure either how much you know about a certain topic or term ending exams (i.e. your achieved knowledge) such as mathematics or spelling, or how much a capacity you have, i.e. your aptitude) to master material in a particular area, such as mechanical relationships.
2. It measured in terms of Individual differences learning of job and skill in doing the work and their achievement. It may high/low with suitable training.

TYPES

Manual Aptitude Test	*Mechanical Aptitude Test*	*Clerical Aptitude Test*	*Aptitude Test Batteries*
Speed and co-ordination of movement. (e.g.) packers, polishers paper folder, cutters, pot makers etc.	Not a single unitary function. It cover variety of factors such as: 1. Spatial visualization 2. Perceptual speed 3. Mechanical Information and 4. Manual dexterity 5. Higher level of organization (e.g. Mechanical relationship, Adjustment, Repair and assembly of machinery)	Indicate 4 different abilities Perceptual –ability to observe words and Numbers. Intellectual ability to groups meaning of words and symbols Various mental skill Add multiply, spell correctly Ability to manipulate with fingers various paper, cards, Typewriter computer	Use for personal selection and vocational study and interpret intra-individual difference DAT- Differential aptitude Test GATB- general Aptitude test Batteries. Diff – verbal Reasoning numerical ability abstract reasoning spatial relationship, mechanical, comprehension, clerical speed accuracy, Language use.

INTELLIGENCE TEST

Intelligence test attempt to measure your intelligence—that is your basic ability to understand the world around you assimilate its functioning and apply this knowledge to enhance the quality of your life.

Classification of intelligence by IQ range

Profound mental retardation	– Below 20 (or) 25
Sever MR	– 20-25 to 35-40
Moderate MR	– 35-40 to 50-55
Mild MR	– 50-55 to about 70
Borderline	– 70-79
Dull Normal	– 80 to 90
Normal	– 90 to 110
Bright Normal	– 110 to 120
Superior	– 120 to 130
Very superior	– 130 and above.

DAVID WECHSLER (1939) Constructed, the best standardized and most widely used intelligence test in clinical practice today. WISC—Wechsler intelligence Scale for children- 5 to 15 yr and WPPSI—Wechsler Preschool and Primary Scale of intelligence- 4 to 6 ½ yr.

WAIS – WECHSLER ADULT INTELLIGENCE SCALE

Subtest: 1. Verbal subtest 6

1. Information
2. Comprehension
3. Arithmetic
4. Similarities
5. Digit span
6. Vocabulary

2. Performance subtest 5

1. Picture completion
2. Block design
3. Picture arrangement
4. Object assembly
5. Digit symbol.

Staford-Binet intelligence scale: In this instrument, Terman used the ratio and mental age to chronological age. This ratio- or quotient- concept led to the use of the term IQ (Intelligence Quotient). IQ = MA/CA × 100.

NEUROPSYCHOLOGICAL TEST

Neuropsychological tests attempt to measure deficits in cognitive functioning (i.e. your ability to think, speak reason etc.) that may result from some sort of brain damage, such as stroke or a brain injury.

Reasoning, Concept Formation and Problem Solving	Wisconsin card scoring test (WCST)	Assesses abstract reasoning and flexibility in problem solving. (Stimulus card of different color, form and number)
Memory Types i. Immediate memory up to 30 seconds after presentation. ii. Recent memory over the past few hours or days. iii. Recent past memory over the last few months. iv. Remote memory events in the distant past	Wechsler memory scale WMS-R, Memory test battery for adults Benton visual retention Test.	It composite of (i) Verbal paired associate and paragraph retention (ii) Visual memory for designs, (iii) orientation (iv) Digit span (v) Role recall of the alphabet (vi) and counting backward. Sensitive to short –term memory.
Orientation	Simple test for orientation Benton visual retention test.	Geometric figure for 10 seconds. Patient attempts to draw. Today's date/month/year/ and time
Perceptual and Perceptuo Motor Performance	Double Simultaneous Stimulation test Bender visual motor Gestalt test for both children and adults (1938 by Lauretta Bender) Complex Visual Discrimination.	To assess Visuoperceptive Visuoconstructive capacity and Somatoperceptual defects by test. Defective capacity for perceptual integration. Nine separate design- print against a white background on a separate card – presented with unlined paper, patient ask to copy each design with the card in front of them. No time limit. i Facial recognition test (Identify photos side view front view shadows ect)
Language	The Boston Diagnostic Aphasia Examination includes a speech rating scale fluency is tested.	To Assess Ideomotor praxis that is symbolic buccofacial and limb movement to exhibit gestures and to demonstrate the use of imagined or real objects.

Contd...

Contd...

Attention and Concentration	Reflects in an oscillation in performance level for a continuous or repeated activity.	Instability in performance variability and speed of simple response.

COMPREHENSIVE TESTING

Neuropsychological test batteries

1. Luria—Nebraska Neuropsychological Battery.
2. Halstead—Reitan Battery of Neuropsychogical test.

Luria-Nebraska Neuropsychological Battery

1. Based on Russian Neuropsychologist Alexander Lusia.
2. To assess a wide range of cognitive functions:
   - Memory
   - Motor function
   - Rhythm
   - Tactile auditory and visual function
   - Receptive and expressive speech
   - Writing
   - Spelling
   - Reading and
   - Arithmetic.

Specific types of problems 15 years and above.

Children's version 8 to 12 years. The test is extremely Sensitive for Identifying.

Halstead-Reitan battery (HRB) of neuropsychological test used to determine the location and effect of specific brain lesions.

OCCUPATIONAL TESTS

It attempt to, match your interests with the interest of persons in known careers. The logic here is, that if the thing that interest you in life match up with, say the thing, that interest most school teachers, then you might make a good school teacher yourself.

PERSONALITY TESTS

It attempt to measure your basic personality style, and are most used in research or forensic setting to help with clinical diagnoses. Two of the most well-known personality tests are:

- ***The Minnesota Multiphasic Personality Inventory (MMPI)***, or the revised MMPI, composed of several hundred "yes or no" questions

Test	*Procedure*	*Measures*
Category Test	Discover the common element in a set of pictures	Concept function Abstraction and Visual acuity
Tactual Performance Test	Place shapes in a form of board while blind folded and then must recall the arrangement of the board.	Dexterity spatial memory and tactual discrimination.
Rhythm Test	Identify 30 pairs of rhythmic beats	Auditory perception attention and Concentration
Finger Oscillation Test	Taps the index finger of each hand in a measured 20 sec period.	Dexterity and motor speed
Speech- sound Perception Test	Matches 60 nonsense syllabus that hear with several printed alternatives	Auditory discrimination and phonetic skills
Trail- making Test	First connects 25 number of circles in order and than connects 25 lettered and number of circle in order (Alternate between numbers and alphabetic.	Vasomotor perception motor speech.
Critical Aflicker Frequency	Notes when flickering lights become steady	Visual perception
Time Serve Test	Judges without looking the time it takes for the second hand of a watch to make several revolutions	Memory and spatial perception
Aphasia Screening Test	Name objects Read write calculate, draw shapes, Identify body parts, difference between relationship	Verbal and non verbal brain functions.
Sensory Perceptual Test	Performs a number of task with eyes closed Identify where and when touch on the hand and face.	Simultaneous stimulation test and tactile perception

- *The Rorschach (the "inkblot test),* composed of several cards of inkblots, you simply give description of the images, and feelings, you experience in looking at the blots.

PERSONALITY TEST

Types

1. Objective, e.g. MMPI, structured clinical.
2. Projective, e.g. Rorschach TAT, SCT word association.

Test	*Type*	*Description*	*Scoring*	*Strengths*
MMPI (Minnesota Multiphase Personality Inventory)	Structured self report or objective test	566 Item checklist true/ false	13 criteria scale	Provides wide range of data on numerous personality values.
Structured Clinical Diagnostic Assessment (Hamilton Rating Scale for Depression)	Semistructured interview Based on DSM IV	--	Numerical 8 scores on diagnostic scales severity of illness monitoring recovery	Assessing the treatment response
Rorschach Ink Blot (Herman Rorschach)	Unstructured project	10 ambiguous ink blots response score on multiple criteria	Accuracy of form location use of color shading ect provide summary scores.	Most widely used interpretative data available
Tat Thematic Perception	'Unstructured project'	20 ambiguous cards depicting a number of scenes	Affects, outcomes and other qualities	Widely used Hands of well Trained person provide valuable information
Sentence Completion Test (Sack)	Structured projective test	A number of devices available all sharing the same formant with more similarities then difference.	Response to half completed sentences.	Brief Administrate time can be useful adjunct to clinical Interviews
Holtzman Ink Blot Test	Unstructured project test	Two parallel forms, of ink blot cards with 45 cards perform	Accuracy of form, location, use of color, etc. Summary score	Only one Response is allowed per card.

INVENTORIES

- Self report—Questionnaire type of personality inventory is the personal data sheet.
- It devised by RS Wood Wart, use in world war I, and published in 1919.
- Questionnaire consists of a list of items, in the form of question, about himself to be answered by the individual.
- It is use to defect personality and behavior symptoms of mal-adjustment.

1. Bell Adjustment Inventory

Question to evaluate the subject status:

Home	*Satisfaction (or) dissatisfaction with home*
Health	*Extent of illness*
Social adjustment	*Extent of shyness/Submissiveness/Intro-version*

Emotional adjustment	*Extent of depression/nervousness/ease of disturbance*
Occupation adjustment	*Satisfaction with work/associative and condition.*

2. Bernreuter Personality Inventory

Question for use in grades 9 to 16 years and with adults.
Score for six traits:

1. Neurotic tendency
2. Self sufficiency
3. Introvesion – extroversion
4. Dominance – submission
5. Confidence
6. Sociability.

3. California Test of Personality

Concept of life adjustment balance between personal and social adjustment.

4. The Minnesota Personality Scale

- Separate forms for men and women.
- Morale/social adjustment/emotional (degree of stability) family relationships/ economic conservation.
- Consist of 550 statements: true/false/cannot say:

The point of view determining important of a trait in that of clinical or personnel worker who wish to assay their Traits.

SPECIFIC CLINICAL TESTS

It attempt of measure specific clinical matters, such as your current level of anxiety or depression.

THERAPEUTIC COMMUNICATION

NURSE–PATIENT RELATIONSHIP

It is an interaction process, in which the nurse fulfills her role, by using her professional knowledge, and skill in such a way, that she is able to help the patient physically, socially, and emotionally. In nursing relataionship refers to connectedness, in interaction, where each person has an effect upon the others.

FACTORS DETERMINING EFFECTIVE NURSE–PATIENT RELATIONSHIP

In the nurse–patient relationship each interaction or encounter is unique because the patient and the nurse are having their own beliefs, values attitudes and behaviors. But some of the factors which can help her to develop an effective relationship are:

1. Self awareness
2. Attitude towards the patient
3. Ability of developing rapport including warmth and genuiness in her approach and empathizing.

GOAL

The nurse help the patient:

1. To cope with present problems.
2. To understand his problem.
3. To understand his active participation in an experience.
4. To identify emerging problems realistically.
5. To find out a new alternative for his or her problem.
6. To try out a pattern of behavior.
7. To communicate.
8. To socialize.
9. To find a meaning in his illness.

PRINCIPLES OF THERAPEUTIC COMMUNICATION

1. Accept the patient exactly as he is.
2. Use self-understanding as a therapeutic tool.
3. Use consistent behaviour to increase patients emotional security.
4. Give reassurance to patients in subtle and acceptable manner.
5. Change patient's behavior through emotional experienance and not by rational interpretation.
6. Avoid unnecessary increase in patients anxiety.
7. Demonstrate objective observation to understand and interpret the meaning of patient's behavior.
8. Maintain realistic nurse-patient relationship.
9. Avoid physical and verbal force as much as possible.
10. Provide nursing care to the patient.
11. Explain routines and procedures at patients level of understanding .
12. Many procedures are modified but basic principles remain unaltered.

PHASES

There are four phases:

1. Pre-interaction phase

2. Introductory or orientation phase
3. Working phase
4. Termination phase.

NURSE TASK IN EACH PHASE OF THE RELATIONSHIP PROCESS

Phase	*Task*
Preinteraction	Explore own feelings, fantasies, and fears. Analyze own professional strengths and limitation Gather data about patient when possible plan for first meeting with patient.
Introductory, or orientation	Determine why patient sought help, Establish trust, acceptance, and open communication Mutually formulate a contract Explore patients thoughts feelings, and action, identify patients problems Define goals with the patient
Working	Explore relevant stressors promote patients development of insight and use of constructive coping mechanisms. Overcome resistance behaviors
Termination	Establish reality of separations Review progress of therapy and attainment of goals Mutually explore feelings of rejection loss, sadness, and anger and related behavior.

THERAPEUTIC COMMUNICATION TECHNIQUES

Technique: Listening

Definition: An active process of receiving information and examining reaction to the messages received.
Example: Maintaining eye contact and receptive nonverbal communication.
Therapeutic value: Nonverbally communicates to the patient the nurse's interest and acceptance.
Nontherapeutic threat: Failure to listen.

Technique: Broad Openings

Definition: Encouraging the patient to select topics for discussion.
Example: "What are you thinking about?"

Therapeutic value: Indicates acceptance by the nurse and the value of the patient's initiative.

Nontherapeutic threat: Domination of the interaction by the nurse; rejecting responses.

Technique: Restating

Definition: Repeating the main thought the patient expressed.

Example: "You say that your mother left you when you were 5 years old."

Therapeutic value: Indicates that the nurse is listening and validates, reinforces, or calls attention to something important that has been said.

Nontherapeutic threat: Lack of validation of the nurse's interpretation of the message; being judgmental; reassuring; defending.

Technique: Clarification

Definition: Attempting to put into words vague ideas or unclear thoughts of the patient to enhance the nurse's understanding or asking the patient to explain what he or she means.

Example: "I'm not sure what you mean. Could you tell me about that again?"

Therapeutic value: Helps to clarify feelings, ideas, and perceptions of the patient and provide an explicit correlation between them and the patient's actions.

Nontherapeutic threat: Failure to probe; assumed understanding.

Technique: Reflection

Definition: Directing back the patient's ideas, feelings, questions, or content.

Example: "You're feeling tense and anxious and it's related to a conversation you had with your husband last night?"

Therapeutic value: Validates the nurse's understanding of what the patient is saying and signifies empathy, interest, and respect for the patient.

Nontherapeutic threat: Stereotyping the patient's responses; inappropriate timing of reflections; inappropriate depth of feeling of the reflections; inappropriate to the cultural experience and educational level of the patient.

Technique: Humor

Definition: The discharge of energy through the comic enjoyment of the imperfect.

Example: "That gives a whole new meaning to the word nervous," said with shared, kidding between the nurse and patient.

Therapeutic value: Can promote insight by making conscious repressed material, resolving paradoxes, tempering aggression, and revealing new options, and is a socially acceptable form of sublimation.

Nontherapeutic threat: Indiscriminate use; belittling patient; screen to avoid therapeutic intimacy.

Technique: Informing

Definition: The skill of information giving.
Example: "I think you need to know more about how your medication works."
Therapeutic value: Helpful in health teaching or patient education about relevant aspects of patient's well-being and self-care.
Nontherapeutic threat: Giving advice.

Technique: Focusing

Definition: Questions or statements that help the patient expand on a topic of importance.
Example: "I think that we should talk more about your relationship with your father."
Therapeutic value: Allows the patient to discuss central issues and keeps the communication process goal directed.
Nontherapeutic threat: Allowing abstractions and generalizations; changing topics.

Technique: Sharing Perceptions

Definition: Asking the patient to verify the nurse's understanding of, what the patient is thinking or feeling.
Example: "You're smiling but I sense that you are really very angry with me."
Therapeutic value: Conveys the nurse's understanding to the patient and has the potential for clearing up confusing communication.
Nontherapeutic threat: Challenging the patient; accepting literal responses; reassuring; testing; defending.

Technique: Theme Identification

Definition: Underlying issues or problems experienced by the patient that emerge repeatedly during the course of the nurse-patient relationship.
Example: "I've noticed that in all of the relationships that you have described, you've been hurt or rejected by the man. Do you think this is an underlying issue?"
Therapeutic value: Allows the nurse to best promote the patient's exploration and understanding of important problems.
Nontherapeutic threat: Giving advice; reassuring; disapproving.

Technique: Silence

Definition: Lack of verbal communication for a therapeutic reason.

Example: Sitting with a patient and nonverbally communicating interest and involvement.

Therapeutic value: Allows the patient time to think and gain insights, slows the pace of the interaction and encourages the patient to initiate conversation, while conveying the nurse's support, understanding, and acceptance.

Nontherapeutic threat: Questioning the patient; asking for "why" responses; failure to break a nontherapeutic silence.

Technique: Suggesting

Definition: Presentation of alternative ideas for the patient's consideration relative to problem solving.

Example: "Have you thought about responding to your boss in a different way when he raises that issue with you? For example, you could ask him whether a specific problem has occurred."

Therapeutic value: Increases the patient's perceived options or choices.

Nontherapeutic threat: Giving advice; inappropriate timing; being judgmental.

CLINICS/CAMPS

INTRODUCTION

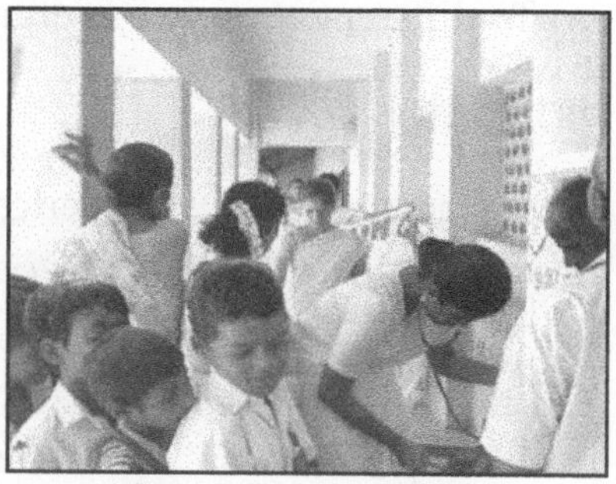

For a long time, psychiatric care was available only in mental hospitals, which were far removed from other hospitals and even cities. One accompaniment of the de-institutionalization of psychiatry was its acceptance in general hospital settings. The next logical step in the same direction was integration of psychiatry in the primary health care. This integration aimed at the application of psychiatric knowledge by the medical and paramedical personnel of the primary health care settings to provide at least basic mental health care.

Applying the broad principles of primary care in the context of mental health

1. Equitable distribution.
2. Preventive approach.
3. Multisectorial efforts.
4. Community participation.

The objectives of rural mental health camps are:

1. To ensure the availability and accessibility of minimum mental health care for all in the foreseeable future, particularly to the most vulnerable and underprivileged sections of populations.
2. To encourage application of mental health knowledge in general health care and in social development.
3. To promote community participation in the mental health service development and to stimulate efforts towards self help in the community.

NARCOANALYSIS

DEFINITION

Narcotherapy refers to Intravenous (Iv) of the drugs, sedatives or stimulants to the patient, as an adjunct to psychotherapy.

HISTORY

Blackwem — Was the first to advocate the IV sodium amytal in psychiatric condition.

Hortey (1926) — Originated the narco analysis which involved the use of both sodium pentothal and sodium amytal.

Purpose — Creation of altered state of awareness or consciousness.

To provide symptomatic relief for severely agitated clients.

To differentiate between organic disabilities from functional syndromes.

INDICATION

Severly agitated clients, hysterical amnesia, suicide case, paranoid illness.

Organic brain syndrome, schizophrenia, depression.

TECHNIQUE

1. Simple catharsis – pentothal interview.
2. Suggestion – suggestion while under the drug.
3. Narcoanalysis and narco synthesis (Both Procedure).

Dose: 2.5 to 5%

Administration: Antecubital vein.

– 5% pentothal solution inj at rate od 2 cc/minute.

(Thiopentone is very short acting barbirate produce unconscious 15-30 sec.)

AVERSION THERAPY

DEFINITION

Aversion therapy is a form of behavior therapy in which an aversive (causing a strong feeling of dislike or disgust) stimulus is paired with an undesirable behavior in order to reduce or eliminate that behavior.

GOAL

- Decrease or eliminate undesirable behaviors
- Treatment focuses on changing a specific behavior itself, unlike insight-oriented approaches that focus on uncovering unconscious motives in order to produce change.

USES OF AVERSION THERAPY

- Habits
- Smoking
- Alcoholism
- Gambling
- Violence
- Homosexuality (historically).

Outpatient or inpatient settings as a self-sufficient **intervention** or as part of a multimodal program. Under some circumstances, aversion therapy may be self administered.

PRECAUTIONS

A variety of aversive stimuli have been used as part of this approach, including chemical and pharmacological stimulants as well as electric shock. Foul odors, nasty tastes, and loud noises have been employed as aversive stimuli somewhat less frequently.

The chemicals and medications generate very unpleasant and often physically painful responses. This type of aversive stimulation, may be risky for persons with heart or lung problems because, of the possibility of making the medical conditions worse.

Aversion treatment that makes use of powerful substances customarily (and intentionally) causes extremely uncomfortable consequences, including nausea and vomiting. These effects may lead to poor compliance with treatment, high dropout rates, potentially hostile and aggressive patients, and public relations problems. Social critics, and members of the general public alike often consider this type of treatment punitive and morally objectionable.

INDIVIDUAL THERAPY

One-to-one Basis

Therapist treats one person at an effectiveness based on patient therapeutic relationship.

TYPES

- Psychoanalysis
- Hypnosis
- Abreaction
- Reality's therapy
- Uncovering and
- Supportive therapy.

PYSCHOANALYSIS

- Developed by Freud.
- Focus primarily on the influence of unconscious forces such as represses impulse memories, internal conflicts and childhood trauma on the mental life and adjustment of the individual.
- Foundation based on problems in early psycho sexual development.
- Oedipus complex—The pleasure and reality principles.
- The system of personality id, ego and super–ego and the important anxiety and defense mechanism against anxiety and neurotic reaction. It is a form of therapy It bring about basic modification in the personality.
- Specific methods used therapeutic relationships to achieve the effect of therapy or free association, dream interpretation, analysis of resistance and defenses used by the patient.
- Working through feelings and experience.
- Every interaction lasts for 45 mint four to five days a week, approximately 3-5 yrs, expensive form of therapy in terms of money and time.

HYPNOSIS OR HYPNOTHERAPY

- Is a superficial or deep trance somnolent state/sleep like
- Induced in patient by suggestion of relaxation and conscious attention on a single object.
- Pt becomes highly suggestible, submissive, and abandons control and response, to therapists influence.
- Induced to recall forgotten events become insensitive to pain gain relief from tension, anxiety, and other psychiatric signs and symptoms.
- It affects behavioral changes and control of attitudes. It is effective in obesity hypertension, asthma, smoking, peptic ulcer, overeating, and other addictive disorder.

ABREACTION

Talks about repressed emotions by reviving and reliving painful experience that they have been buried in the unconscious. Iv of a drug such, as 'pentothal'.

REALITY THERAPY

- Focuses on the present behavior and development of a patient, ability to cope with the stress of reality, and take a greater responsibility for the fulfillment of his need.
- Therapist involve in active relationship, rejects unrealistic behavior.
- Teaches better way to meet his needs in the real world.
- The patient need to be stressed, past cannot change.
- He must take response of wright/wrong action of the present.

Uncovering or Insight Psychotherapy

- To break the patients repressed conflicts and traumatic experience to the surface.
- It helps the patient in gainning an 'Insight'.
- Patient explores different methods to cope with the problem once he gains an insight into his conflict or problem.

SUPPORTIVE PSYCHOTHERAPY

Surface Therapy

1. Mental ventilation
2. Environmental modification changing the living condition
3. Persuasion to modify the family behavior mother (e.g.) neglect girl child
4. Reeducation problems
5. Reassurance there are possibility of improvement.

GROUP THERAPY

DEFINITION

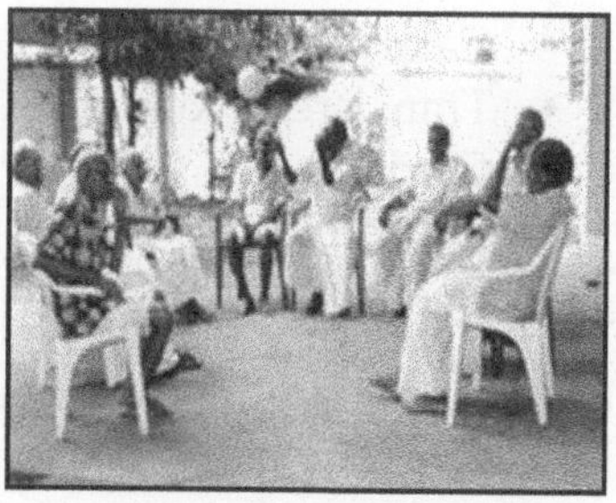

Group psychotherapy is a treatment of psychological problems in which two or more patient interact with each other, on both an emotional and cognitive levels in the presence of one or more psychotherapists.

INDICATIONS

- Alcoholism
- Obesity
- Drug addiction.

TYPES

1. Traditional groups
2. Encounter groups or T – Group
3. Homogenous or heterogonous groups
4. Open or close groups
5. Groups for psycho's or neurosis.

STEPS OF GROUP THERAPY

1. Developing contact in group
2. Selecting the members in group
3. Selection of group leaders.

TECHNIQUES

1. 8 to 10 persons involved in group
2. 1 to 2 hours session.
   (Session are held once or twice a week)

APPROACHES

1. Psychoanalysis
2. Supportive therapy
   — Ventilation
   — Reassurance
   — Reeducation
3. Transactional analysis
4. Behavior therapy.

ROLE OF NURSE

- Catalyst
- Transference object
- Clarifier
- Interpreter
- Role model and resource person
- Supporter

FAMILY THERAPY

DEFINITION

It is that branch of psychotherapy that sees an Individual Psychiatric symptoms to the family in which he lives.

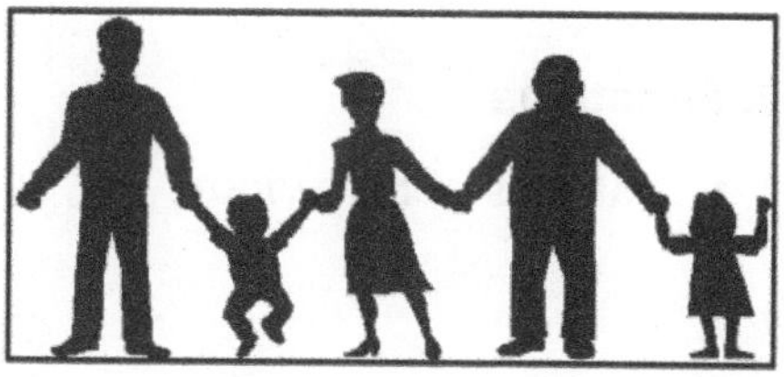

COMPONENTS OF A FAMILY ASSESSMENT

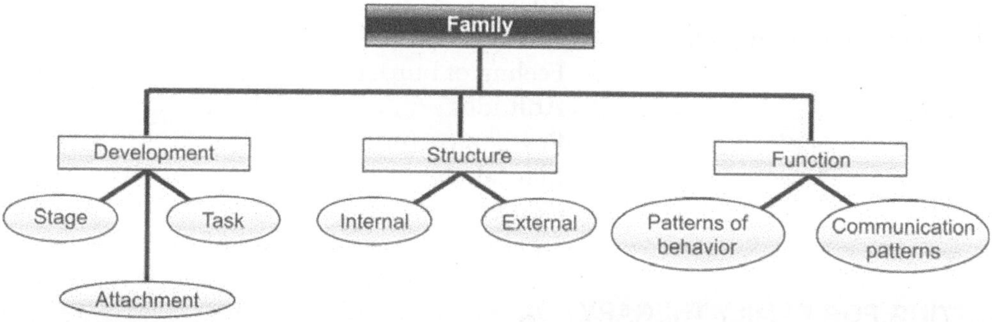

1. Development

- Stage
  - Transition points
  - Appropriate or
  - In appropriate affect
- Attachment
  - Functional
  - Dysfunctional
- Task
  - Status
  - Task fulfillment
  - Task failure

2. Structure

- External
  - Extended family
  - Culture
  - Religion
  - Community
  - Social class
  - Education.
- Internal
  - Hierarchical structure
  - Household composition
  - Boundaries

- Sibling subsystem
- Rank order

3. Functions

- Patterns of Behaviour
  - Level of differentiation
  - Alliances
  - Strengths
  - Coping style
  - Daily routine
  - Task allocation
  - Roles.
- Communication patterns
  - Triangle
  - Feeling of burden
  - Attitudes
  - Power structure
  - Marital reciprocity
  - Conflict resolution
  - Family

SETTING FOR FAMILY THERAPY

1. Community base office
2. In patient units before discharge
3. Home.

TECHNIQUES

1. Focusing on here and now interactions
2. Restructuring family interactional patterns
3. Classifying communication
4. Reframing
5. Challenging the client.

APPROACHES

1. Family communication is open and direct.
2. Family resolve conflicts effectively.
3. Family members enact roles flexibly and effectively.
4. Problem solving skills are evident.
5. Anxiety and stress are managed through use of effective coping skills.
6. Family power structure reflects balanced influence and control.
7. Family members demonstrate functional interactional pattern.

TEAM AND QUALIFICATIONS

1. Psychologist
2. Psychiatric social workers
3. Psychiatric Nurses. Who have completed graduate programme in Family Therapy

ROLE OF NURSE

1. Role model.
2. An educator.
3. Assessing the role assumed by various members of the family.
4. Involving family communication patterns.
5. Achieving the developmental tasks of the family.
6. Normal coping strategies used by the family.
7. Encouraging to family support system.
8. Importance to sociocultural norms and values of the family.

OCCUPATIONAL THERAPY

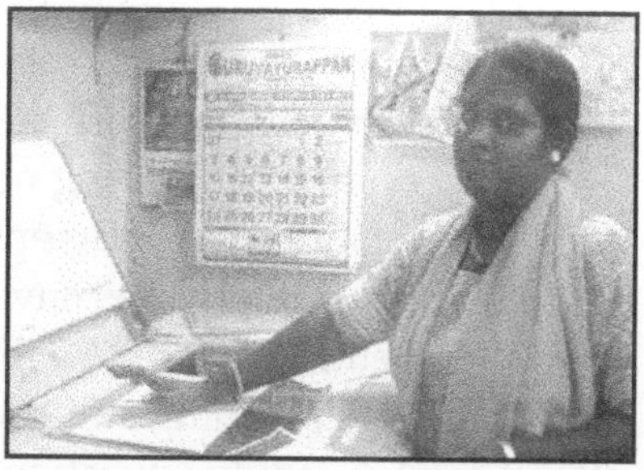

DEFINITION

Occupational therapy is defined as" any activity which engages a persons resources of time and energy and is composed of skills and valves.

— Reed and Sanderson, 1980

GOAL

1. Assess the patient need in terms of occupational role.
2. Identify the skills needed to support those roles.
3. To remove or to minimize behavior that, interfere with occupational performance.
4. To improve role performance.
5. To develop level of competence that will allow satisfactory performance occupational roles.

PROCESS OF INTERVENTION (SEVEN STAGES)

1. Initial evaluation.
2. Development of immediate and long term goals.
3. Development theory plan.
4. Implement the plan.
5. Call for review meeting.
6. Further goal and alter the treatment programme.
7. Recording.

AREAS OF THERAPY

1. Basic skills simple task performance.
2. Group participation.
3. Other skills self care domestic work.
4. Recreation.
5. Productive work.
6. Intimacy.

APPROACHES

1. Work-oriented activities.
2. Recreational.
3. Creative expressive activities.
4. Group or individual therapy.

TYPES OF SERVICE

1. Independent living skills—Self-care or self maintenance.
2. Task oriented treatment using creativity in crafts, education, leisure time, play, socialization and other role related activities.
3. Provocational and work adjustment program.
4. Sensory motor including neuromuscular assessment and treatment.
5. Design fabrication and application of orthotic devices.
6. Adaptation to physical environment and guidance in use of adaptive equipment.
7. Therapeutic exercise to enhance functional performance.
8. Discharge planning and community reentry.
9. Patient or family education and counseling.

SETTING

1. Institutional – Psychiatric hospitals and nursing homes.
2. Community based partial hospitalization.
3. Residential treatment.
4. Forensic program.
5. Psychosocial and physical rehabilitation centers.
6. Special school for physically and mentally handicapped.
7. Integrated school and community groups homes.
8. Community mental health centers.
9. Day care centers.
10. Industrial health unit.
11. Half way homes.
12. De-addiction centers.

CLASSIFICATION OF OCCUPATIONAL THERAPY (THREE GROUPS)

1. **Diversional therapy**
   - Organizing games which stimulate spontaneity and freedom of movement and the competitiveness and excitement, tends to take away the patient's anxious preoccupation with the disease patient.
2. **Remedial therapy**
   - Include 'physiotherapy' for particular muscle groups (e.g. basket making, carpentry, embroidery, and gardening).
3. **Physiotherapy**
   - Which includes heat massage, electro-therapy, remedial exercise either assisted by the therapist or free or resisted by weights, pulleys, etc.

ROLE OF NURSE

1. Prepare the patient for therapy, and assist the therapist to administer therapies.
2. Take care of the patients after the therapies are overed.
3. Finds opportunity to give group and Individual Health education.
4. Keep link between patients their families, and with the therapist.
5. Co-ordinates the Nursing service with psychosocial therapies.

PSYCHOTHERAPY

DEFINITION

According to Wolberg psychotherapy is a method of treatment based on the development of an intimate relationship between client and the therapist for the purpose of exploring and modifying the clients behavior in a satisfying direction.

GOAL

1. To change maladaptive behavior.
2. To remove or reduce the factors causing distinct behavior.
3. To grow and develop coping mechanism.
4. To solve problem in future.
5. To improve in social function.
6. To develop self-confidence.
7. Helping patient to resolve inner conflicts.

TYPES

1. Simple psychotherapy (individual)
2. Supportive psychotherapy (couple)

3. Special methods:
   a. Small groups therapy, bnehavior therapy
   b. Large group therapy.

COMMON FACTORS

1. Listening and talking
2. Restoration of morale
3. Release of emotion
4. Rationale
5. Transference and counter-transference.

PHASES

I – Introductory Phase
II – Working phase
III – Termination phase

NURSES ROLE

1. Assessment and Identify the aspects of problem.
2. Emphasize the patient will helped to find his own solution to his problems.
3. Encourage problem solving methods.
4. Encourage patient to consider alternative ways of thinking.
5. Stimulate the patient to point out any patterns of behaviors.
6. Involve in recreational and relaxation activities.
7. Develop a sense of self identity and self confidence.

MILIEU THERAPY

Milieu is a french word derived from:

- *Mi* means " middle".
- *Lieu* means "place".

So milieu means environment or settings.

Therapeutic milieu means providing a health environment which helps in the recovery of the patient.

" Therapeutic community "is a term applied by the English psychiatrist Maxwell Jones (1953).

DEFINITION

Milieu therapy or Therapeutic Community approach attempts to make the maximum use of:

i. The social system and its constituents with patients, his relatives and neighbours.
ii. Personnel and the hospital community (i.e., psychiatrist, nurse, psychologist, social worker, other patients).
iii. To modify the patients behavior so that he may manage his life and his personal relationship in a more constructive manner.

GOALS

1. To minimize the anti therapeutic environment.
2. To minimize prolongation of hospitalization by helping in early recovery.
3. To minimize maladaptive behaviors, creating an environment, where maladaptive behavior is discouraged.
4. To provide a free and favorable climate.
5. To help the patient to improve his self esteem.

PRINCIPLES

1. Group activity approach.
2. Democracy help in increasing the self-respect of a patient.
3. Patient is involved in his own therapy, which helps him in making decision.
4. Decision making ability improve the self confidence of patients.
5. It provides an environment of free communication.
6. Direct his focus of attention not only on his own need but also on other need.
7. It reduces social isolation and dehumanization.

IMPORTANT ASPECTS

- Governing system.
- Communication is open and free.
- Goals are increase self esteem, decrease hospital stay, and anti therapeutic environment.
- Therapeutic community is placed on social and group intervention.

TEAM

Psychiatrist

Psychiatric nurse

Psychologist

Technical staff

Support personal.

ROLE OF NURSE

Tripartite Role

1. Authoritarian Role – Control the group and set limits.
2. Social role – Encourages and support in various ways communication discussion and talking to the team members.
3. Therapeutic Role – By giving medicine, Therapeutic Relationship, Making observation and reporting.

BEHAVIOR THERAPY

DEFINITION

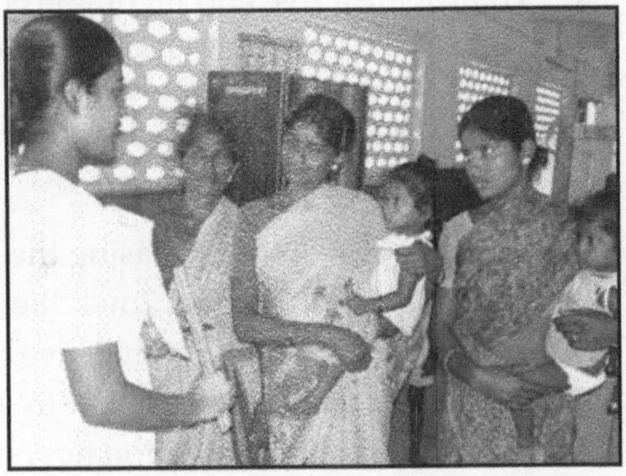

Behavior therapy is any observable, recordable and measurable act. Movement or response of individual. at changing maladaptive behavior.

GOAL

1. To increase activity
2. To reduce unwanted behavior
3. To increase pleasure
4. Enhancing social skills.

PRINCIPLES

a. Behavior analysis
b. Graduated approach
c. Experimental format:
Classical conditioning—Pavlov
Operant conditioning—Skinner.

PHASES

1. Antecedent 2. Behavior 3. Consequence

1. **Antecedent phase**
   - Assessment
   - Collecting information
   - Identify and defining the problem.

2. **Behavior phase**
   - Action or series of step
   - Discrete action.
3. **Consequence phase**
   - What kind of effect (positive, negative or neutral effect)
   - Identify the Environment Variable that influence.

Affective – Emotion or feeling.

Behavior – Outward manifestation and action.

Cognitive – thought about situation.

INDICATIONS

- Agoraphobia
- Alcohol dependence
- Anorexia nervosa
- Bulimia nervosa
- Phobia
- Paraphilia
- Schizophrenia
- Sexual dysfunction
- Desensitization
- Obesity
- Cocaine dependence
- Chronic nightmare
- Compulsion
- Psychosomatic
- Smoking
- Tension.

TECHNIQUES

1. Shaping
2. Modeling
3. Premack principle
4. Extinction
5. Contingency contracting
6. Token economy
7. Time out
8. Reciprocal inhibition
9. Overt sensitization
10. Covert sensitization

11. Desensitization
12. Flooding.

ROLE OF NURSE

- As educator
- Counselor
- Advice
- Co-ordinator and facilitator.

RELAXATION THERAPY

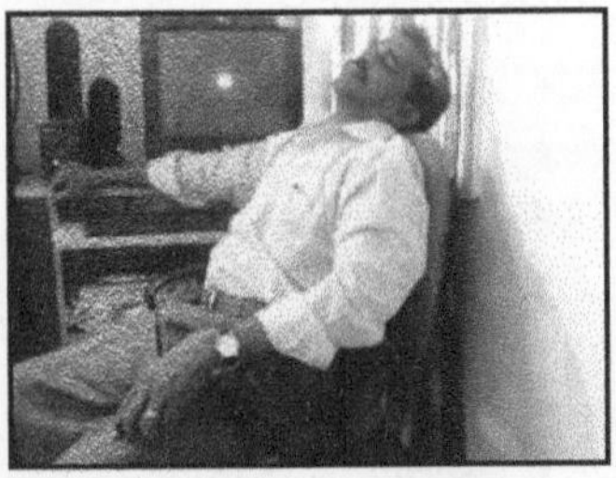

Relaxation: A state of relative freedom from both anxiety and skeletal muscle tension.

The Specific Effects Model

The frequently observed desynchronies across behavioral, cognitive, and somatic measures of anxiety has led researchers (e.g., Davidson and Schwartz, 1976) to develop the specific-effects model.

The Relaxation Response Model

H. Benson (1975, 1983), based in his observation of the relaxation effects, argued that all the relaxation techniques produce a single "relaxation response," characterized by diminished sympathetic arousal.

Integrative Model

Schwartz, Davidson, and Goleman (1978), suggests that the majority of the relaxation procedures have highly specific effects, as well as more generally stress-reducing effects, therefore, the specific effects of various relaxation techniques may be superimposed upon a general relaxation effect.

Some ideas on how to pace yourself

1. **Keep a simple diary of everything you do** for at least two weeks. Write down how you felt at mid-day, at tea-time and at bed-time. You can get someone to help you do this if you find it hard to remember or if you feel too tired.
2. After two weeks, read over it, to find out what things you did easily without getting tired. **You may find you ought to start doing less!**
3. Carry on keeping your diary.
4. When you read your diary you may spot that, **certain things you did made you very tired**, like having to do a lot of talking. Could it be that phone calls are a real problem for you? Check.
5. Mental tasks, like **talking and listening, can be very tiring**. So, when thinking about things to do, it is important to include **thinking tasks**, such as reading and

writing, as well as those that are **physical**, such as brushing your teeth or getting dressed. Most of the things, we do need to use both brain and muscle power.

6. Quite often the full effect of something you did won't be felt for **up to 3 days afterwards**. A diary can be really helpful in spotting these sorts of patterns.
7. **Don't just do things the way you have always done them**. For example, if you get up in the morning, and eat your breakfast, maybe have a rest before you get dressed.
8. If you get tired in the middle of doing something - **STOP!** Go back to it later in the day or week.
9. As the days and weeks go by, try to **build up slowly**. Little by little you do more and more. You may have set-backs and off-days, but that is normal. **Don't push too hard**.
10. Your muscles may ache at times. This is normal if you haven't used those muscles for a while. But watch out! Really bad aches or pain mean you are pushing too hard. Don't do it. **Pace yourself!** You have to **become an expert at reading your body**.
11. **Do more of the sort of things you enjoy and are good at**, so that you are less likely to get fed up or bored and give up.
12. It can really help to **switch between brain activities**, like reading and listening, and moving about, physical activities.
13. Make sure you make time to **rest and relax**. Resting means just that - doing nothing! Reading and watching TV may be relaxing, but your brain will still be active. Sit in a comfy chair or lie down. Why not listen to a tape or CD that is especially made to help people relax?
14. **Don't be tempted to compare what you can do now with what you used to do before you got ill**. It will make you really fed up and gets you nowhere!
15. Many people find that they **begin to feel better as soon as they stop fighting the illness**. Do what you can. Build up gently. In the end the illness will have run its course and you will have helped yourself to get strong again.

YOGA AND MENTAL HEALTH

Those practicing yoga experiences a number of factors that results in a profound effect on their mental health. These can be classified under:

1. Reduction of tension and
2. Rrestoration of pliability.
3. "Personal" and
4. "Social."

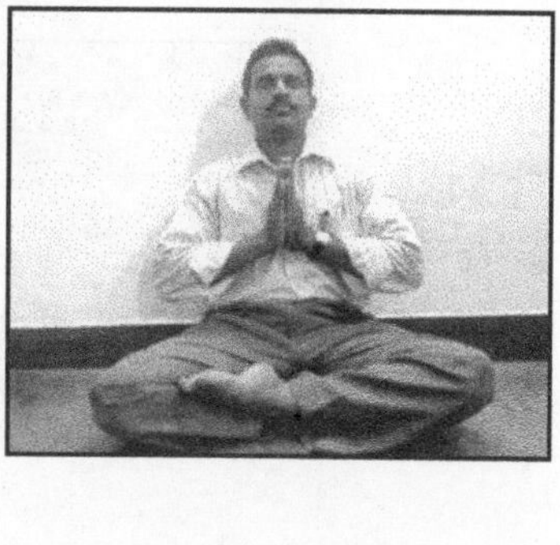

1. REDUCTION OF TENSION

Many people who practice yoga speak of "freeing the mind from mental disturbances," "calming the spirit," or "steadying the mind." Reduction of nervousness, irritability and confusion, depression and mental fatigue are some of the benefits experienced. One experiences a relief from the pressure of his "compulsions." His nervousness, especially any jitteriness, should subside or disappear.

2. RESTORATION OF PLIABILITY

"The positive side of the benefits from a full round of yogic exercises may be described as renewal of mental agility. Both mood and capacity for alertness, attentiveness and willingness to tackle problems revive. One may not be able to rekindle boundless enthusiasm late in a working day; early morning, or even noonday, efforts to recharge mental energies can revive a full measure of willingness.

3. PERSONAL VALUES

a. **Avoidance of fear**: Yoga is said to result in the reduction of a variety of **mental ills.** These may range all the way from vague feelings of frustration, persecution, insecurity, on the one hand, to acute and specific types of insanity, on the other.
b. **Acceptance of faith in life.** The goal of yoga is confident living. Its aim is to replace pessimism and its varieties such as cynicism with a "Yea-saying" appreciation of life, not only on any given day, but as a gracious, wonderful whole. When you achieve the yogic spirit, then you can say with the Stoics, "I accept the universe.

4. SOCIAL VALUES

a. Yoga may reduce your annoyance with others and others' annoyance with you. If you become less irritable, you tend to irritate others less and tend to be less irritated by what others do when they present themselves as problems to you.
b. You tend to be easier to get along with and you tend to find others easier to get along with.

RECREATIONAL THERAPY

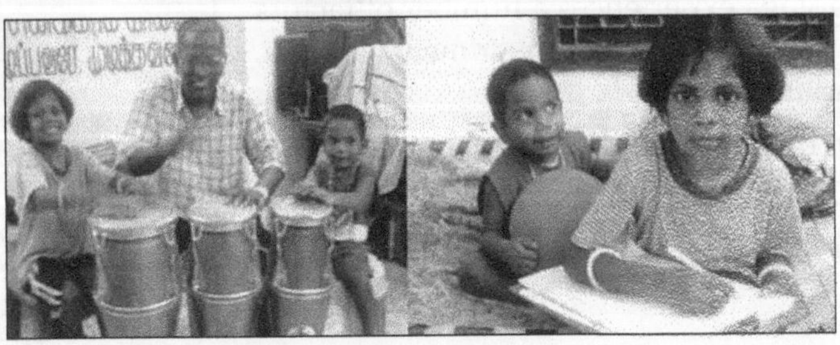

Recreation therapy, also referred to as **recreational therapy** and **therapeutic recreation**, contributes to the broad spectrum of health care through treatment, education, and the provision of adapted recreational opportunities—all of which aid in improving and maintaining physical, cognitive, emotional, and social functioning, preventing secondary health conditions, enhancing independent living skills and overall quality of life.

DEFINITION

It is a form of activity therapy, where an individual enjoys pleasurably, leisure time through recreating and renewing the body and mind by relieving emotional tension or internal conflicts and thereby releases monotonus life of mentally ill person.

Treatment services utilize leisure activities to diminish or eliminate disabling conditions.

These conditions may include physical, cognitive, social, emotional, spiritual, or other areas which limit the individual.

The recreational therapist may use a variety of techniques, including arts and crafts:

- Animals,
- Sports,
- Games,
- Dance and movement,
- Drama,
- Music, and
- Community reintegration outings.

A recreational therapist works with the client, their family members and other close friends to improve their health condition.

Recreation Therapists provide a variety of interventions

- Leisure counselling
- Values clarification
- Bibliotherapy
- Cinematherapy
- Horticulture therapy
- Therapeutic community
- Humor
- Therapeutic use of touch
- Relaxation techniques
- Physical activity

- Aromatherapy
- Assertiveness training
- Social skills training
- Cognitive rehabilitation
- Animal-assisted therapy
- Aquatic therapy
- Creative arts
- Reality orientation
- Validation therapy
- Remotivation
- Resocialization
- Sensory training
- Self-esteem training and reminiscence.

Leisure education is aimed at providing clients with information to help return to a meaningful leisure lifestyle.

This may include information related to topics such as adapted sports, motivational techniques, implementing healthy and active lifestyles, leisure availability, community programs, transportation options, support networks, and appropriate leisure options to drugs and alcohol abuse.

ROLE OF NURSE

- Plan the recreational activities based on abilities/strengths.
- Encourage to participate in activity.
- Teach the necessary skill for each activity.
- Avoid competitive games.
- Encourage the client to express self.
- Supervise the activity and appreciate the effective performance.
- Settings.
- Acute care hospitals.
- Rehabilitation centers.
- Nursing homes.
- Psychiatric hospitals.
- Community recreation centers.
- Pediatric hospitals.
- Group homes.
- Senior centers.
- Community health centers.
- Public and private schools.

ANIMAL-ASSISTED THERAPY

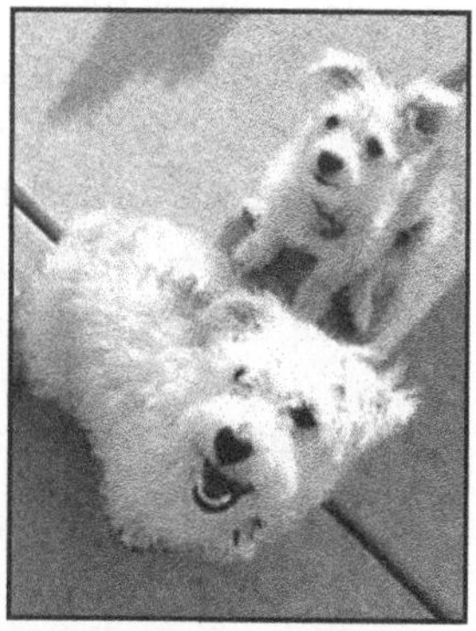

DEFINITION

Animal-assisted therapy is a goal-oriented therapy. It is a structured form where the goals are pre-determined and where the interaction with the animals leads to the goal. When it is structured and goal oriented, it is called animal assisted therapy. But when there are no specific goals other than recreation and it is casual then it is called animal assisted activity.

TYPES

- There are several different kinds of animals used for the therapy process but the most common one is a dog because it is easily trainable, it is more interactive and social.
- Dogs work on their auditory and olfactory senses more. These qualities are worked upon during training.
- Several other animals are used in therapy like cats, birds, and rabbits.
- This is a specialized form of animal assisted therapy. It is mainly used with people who have a physical disability, spastic and autistic children.

(The main focus here is to regain body balance, motor control, and self-esteem).

The kind of animal used differs from setting to setting.

For example, in a geriatric setting, one cannot use a very jumpy or excited dog. Probably in that setting, a cat or a rabbit is more suitable. The individuals can just keep them on their laps and pet. But if it were a children's setting, a dog would be more appropriate. The choice of animals depends on the clients as well as the setting.

Animal-assisted therapy has wide applications in mental health:

1. **Depression** – It helps to build self-esteem. Animals have a non-judgmental attitude and listen willingly to the individual. They show unconditional love and support and also it is easier to open up to an animal.
2. **Hyperactivity** – Playing with animals, especially jumpy dogs, is a good outlet for children's energy. But at the same time it is systematically controlled. The focus in therapy is to increase the attention span and concentration. Normally, hyperactive children cannot sustain at any activity for too long but using this form of therapy, their sustainability at any activity can be increased. It has also been proven that when you pet an animal, your system automatically calms down. It also works with people who have high blood pressure.
3. **Autism** – Children with autism lack social skills, communication, and cannot relate to human beings. But they interact extremely well with animals. It is very hard to neglect an animal when in a therapy room.

4. **Stress** – Animals help to reduce stress. Research has shown that watching a fish tank helps reduce your stress and brings down the blood pressure.
5. **Mental retardation, cerebral palsy and spastic children behavioral problems** – These days, a lot of parents come in with behavioral complaints of their children. Animal assisted therapy works very well using behavioral techniques.
6. **Reading and learning difficulties** - animal assisted reading has increased popularity and has shown good results.

Animal-assisted therapy is becoming popular form of therapy

- It works as an excellent icebreaker and provides a valuable breakthrough.
- Helps to build rapport.
- Helps in building and improving communication skills.
- It can be incorporated with any other kind of therapy. Works as an excellent co-therapy and enhances the results.
- Lowers anxiety, guards, or defenses.
- Strong motivational point (especially with people having speech disability) very effective with withdrawn or uncommunicative children.

BENEFITS OF ANIMAL-ASSISTED THERAPY

- Rapport building is easier.
- Keeps the focus on the outer world. The animal helps as a link or medium of achieving the goals.
- The animals accept unconditionally and give love irrespective of who the person is. They have an unconditional and non-judgmental attitude and accept the person without any qualifications.
- Help in the socialization process and encourage interaction.
- Helps brighten the atmosphere in an institutional setting, gives mental stimulation, and increases laughter, amusement, and play.
- Physical contact and touch is comforting and therapeutic.
- Through interaction with animals, children learn to be empathetic.
- Working with animals has several physiological benefits as well like reducing stress, anxiety, and blood pressure.
- It provides entertainment in an otherwise routine and monotonous schedule.

THE AREAS THAT ANIMAL-ASSISTED THERAPY WORKS TOWARDS ARE

- *Behavioral*
- *Motivational*
- *Physical*
- *Educational*

- Animal assisted therapists work in collaboration with rehab professionals.
- There are several different therapists involved like physiotherapists, speech therapists, counselors, and other professionals.

The problem areas are identified and an outline of a schedule is made.

The therapist, co-therapist (animal), and client work together towards the goal.

pre-therapy, mid-therapy, and post-therapy evaluations are done.

There is a need to increase awareness about animals.

People should be educated about animals, not just from a therapy point of view but how to co-exist with animals in our environment. People in the urban areas are gradually becoming aversive towards living in the natural environment.People in the rural areas have some or the other domestic animal in their house.

Thus, it works as a therapeutic environment even though it is not as structured as a therapeutic setting.

MUSIC THERAPY

(Music Therapy - "For - Brain, Body and Soul")

Music has frequently been used as a therapeutic agent from the ancient times. Music is a kind of yoga system through the medium of sonorous sound, which acts upon the human organism and awakens and develops their proper functions to extent of self-realisation.

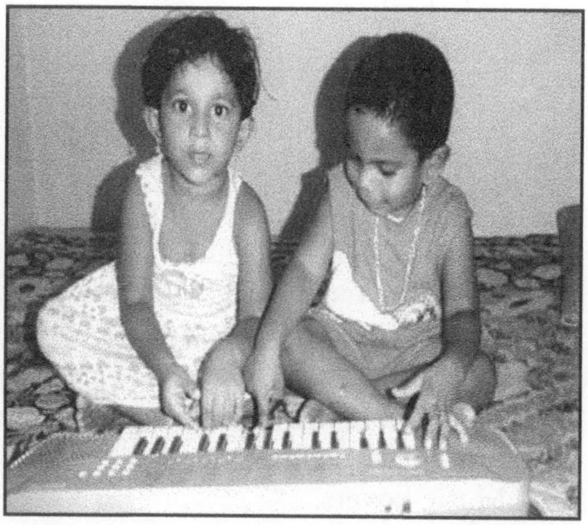

This is the ultimate goal of Hindu Philosophy and religion. Melody is the keynote of Indian Music. The 'Raga' is the basis of melody. Various 'Ragas', have been found to be very effective in curing many diseases.

AIMS OF MUSIC THERAPY

- One obvious use of music is that of a sedative.
- It can replace the administration of tranquilizers, or at least reduce the dosage of tranquillizers.
- Music increases the metabolic activities within the human body.
- It accelerates the respiration, influences the internal secretion, improves the muscular activities and as such affects the Central Nervous System and Circulatory System of the listener and the performer.
- The effect of Music Therapy may be immediate or slow, depending upon number of factors like the subject, his mental condition, environment and the type of Music, selected for having the desired effect.

- Music Therapy largely depends on individual needs and taste.
- The use of Music as therapy is based on scientific and clinical approach and has to be used with great care and deep study of the nature of illness.
- We can call it "The study of Individual- Modality Theory".

Before using music as Therapy it must be ascertained which type of music is to be used?

The concept of Music Therapy is dependent on correct intonation and right use of the basic elements of music.Such as notes [swara] rhythm, volume, beats and piece of melody.

There are countless 'Ragas' of course with countless characteristic peculiarities of their own.That is why we cannot establish a particular Rag for a particular disease. Different types of Ragas are applied in each different case.

When we use term Music Therapy, we think world -wide system of therapy.

INDICATIONS

- Aphasia.
- Developmental disorder.
- Elderly clients.
- Confusion.
- Agitation.
- Affective, cognitive, and sensory disorder.
- Terminally ill patients.

We should apply the formula of three ' Ps ' –

i. **Perfect Time** - It includes duration, span, interval and time to play the music.
ii. **Perfect Direction** - It includes posture and conditions to listen the music.
iii. **Perfect Force** - It includes tone, timber, sound quality, and volume of meditative music.

We should remember the three categories of patient's i.e.

i. Music-Learned,
ii. Music-Lovers,
iii. Non-Musical.

Select the Meditative Music accordingly. Music helps in the treatment of actual diseases in the following manner.

One obvious use of music is that of a sedative. It can replace the administration of tranquilizers, or at least reduce the dosage of tranquilizers. Music increases the metabolic activities within the human body. It accelerates the respiration, influences the internal secretion, improves the muscular activities and as such affects the "Central Nervous System and Circulatory System of the listener and the performer.

(India's First Music Therapist Dr. Bhaskar Khandekar)

BENEFITS OF MUSIC THERAPY

1. Music acts on our mind before being transformed into thought and feeling.
2. Music influences the lower and higher cerebral centers of the brain.
3. Use of Music as a therapy helps search of an individual's personal harmony.
4. Music therapy is an important tool in the treatment of both psychological and psychosomatic disorders.
5. Music Therapy stimulates good vibrations in the nerves of the listeners.
6. Music brings about a sense of mental well being in individuals.
7. Music Therapy helps to clear the junked thought in mind, which leads to have positive frame of mind.
8. Music Therapy enhances the concentration level of children.
9. Music improves the capacity of planning.
10. Music training helps to express refined exhibition of emotions and clarity in cognition too.

Music therapy can be conducted in places like

- Labor room.
- Operating room.
- Massage therapy.
- Counseling hall.
- Rehabilitation center.
- Addiction center.
- Physical therapy units.

PLAY THERAPY

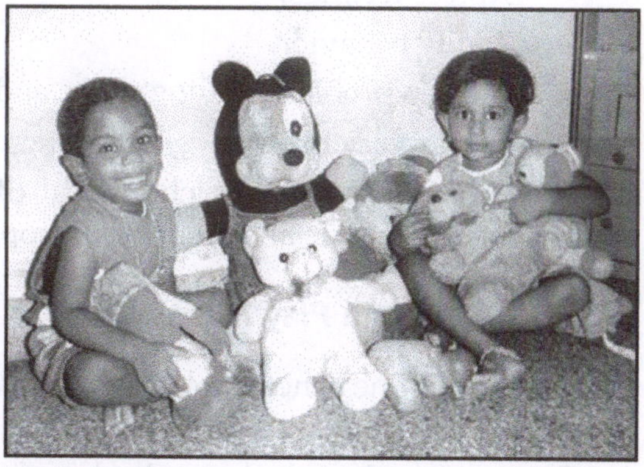

Play therapy as "the systematic use of a theoretical model to establish an interpersonal process wherein trained play therapists use the therapeutic powers of play to help clients prevent or resolve psychosocial difficulties and achieve optimal growth and development."

Play is a fun, enjoyable activity that elevates our spirits and brightens our outlook on life.

It expands self-expression, self-knowledge, self-actualization and self-efficacy.

Play relieves feelings of stress and boredom, connects us to people in a positive way, stimulates creative thinking and exploration, regulates our emotions, and boosts our ego.

In addition, play allows us to practice skills and roles needed for survival.

(Learning and development are best fostered through play).

Why Play in Therapy?

Play therapy is a structured, theoretically based approach to therapy that builds on the normal communicative and learning processes of children.

The curative powers inherent in play are used in many ways.

Therapists strategically utilize play therapy to help children express, what is troubling them when they do not have the verbal language to express their thoughts and feelings.

In play therapy, toys are like the child's words and play is the child's language.

Through play, therapists may help children learn more adaptive behaviors, when there are emotional or social skills deficits.

The positive relationship that develops between therapist and child during play therapy sessions provides a corrective emotional experience necessary for healing.

Play therapy may also be used to promote cognitive development and provide insight about and resolution of inner conflicts or dysfunctional thinking in the child.

What is Play Therapy

Play therapy builds on the natural way that children learn about themselves and their relationships in the world around them.

Through play therapy:

- Children learn to communicate with others,
- Express feelings,
- Modify behavior,
- Develop problem-solving skills, and
- Learn a variety of ways of relating to others.

Play provides a safe psychological distance from their problems and allows expression of thoughts and feelings appropriate to their development.

Who Benefits from Play Therapy?

Although everyone benefits, play therapy is especially appropriate for children ages 3 through 12 years old.

Teenagers and adults have also benefited from play techniques and recreational processes.

To that end, use of play therapy with adults within mental health, agency, and other healthcare contexts is increasing.

In recent years, play therapy interventions have also been applied to infants and toddlers.

How Will Play Therapy Benefit A Child?

Play therapy is implemented as a treatment of choice in mental health, school, agency, developmental, hospital, residential, and recreational settings, with clients of all ages.

Play therapy treatment plans have been utilized as the primary intervention or as an adjunctive therapy for multiple mental health conditions and concerns, e.g., anger management, grief and loss, divorce and family dissolution, and crisis and trauma.

For modification of behavioral disorders, e.g., anxiety, depression, attention deficit hyperactivity (ADHD), autism or pervasive developmental, academic and social developmental, physical and learning disabilities, and conduct disorders.

Play Therapy Helps Children

- Become more responsible for behaviors and develop more successful strategies.
- Develop new and creative solutions to problems.
- Develop respect and acceptance of self and others.
- Learn to experience and express emotion.
- Cultivate empathy and respect for thoughts and feelings of others.
- Learn new social skills and relational skills with family.
- Develop self-efficacy and thus a better assuredness about their abilities

How Long Does Play Therapy Take?

- Each play therapy session varies in length but usually last about 30 to 50 minutes.
- Sessions are usually held weekly.
- Research suggests that it takes an average of 20 play therapy sessions to resolve the problems of the typical child referred for treatment.
- Of course, some children may improve much faster while more serious or ongoing problems may take longer to resolve.

TYPES OF PLAY THERAPY

- Individual play therapy.
- Group play therapy.
- Free play therapy –Freedom to choose the toys or play activity.
- Controlled play therapy-In clinical setting.
- Structured play therapy- Play situation will be organized.
- Un Structured play therapy—Pre planed situation.
- Directive play—Play situation will be created.
- Non-directive play—No direction free of choice.

Who Practices Play Therapy?

The practice of play therapy requires extensive specialized education, training, and experience.

A play therapist is a licensed (or certified) mental health professional, who has earned a Master's or Doctorate degree in a mental health field with considerable general clinical experience and supervision.

With advanced, specialized training, experience, and supervision, mental health professionals may also earn the "Registered Play Therapist (RPT)" or "Registered Play Therapist-Supervisor".

Chapter 8

COUNSELING PATIENT AND FAMILY

DEFINITION

Counseling is emotional intellectual, spiritual and psychological support. It is an implementation method that helps the client use a problem, solving process to recognize and manage stress and that facilitates interpersonal relationships among the client, family and health care team.

—**Patricia A Potter**

STAGES

Stage I—Contact between client and counselor

Stage II—Understanding the problems

Stage III—Knowing measures taken by client to solve the problem.

DO'S AND DONT'S WHILE CONDUCTING INTERVIEW

1. Maintain eye to eye contact
2. Interrupt only, when necessary
3. Ask always open ended questions
4. Do not be hurry
5. Do not pass judgments
6. Do not threaten
7. Don't be little
8. Be reassuring and supportive
9. Clarify
10. Give time
11. Prepare
12. Recording.

MODEL OF COUNSELING

REDA Model

- R – RAPPORT
- E – EXPLORATION

D – DECISION

A – ACTION

	Aim	*Task*	*Skill*	*Activity*
R	Cooperative working relationship	• Welcoming • Introducing • Confidentiality	Attention giving	Confirming contracting
E	To Identify the of the problem. nature	• Obtaining a complete picture of the problem. • Identify most pressing factor. • Understanding the client's general situation.	Asking and leading questions (Opened or closed end)	• Check • Communication • Empathy • Paraphrasing • Summarizing • Focusing
D	Assist the client to make decision	• Introducing different ways of looking at the problem. • Providing new and relevant information	• Client feels, says, does, or believes. • Information giving.	Encouraging and support.
A	To assist the client to plan a course of action and reviewing	• Identifying an appropriate course of action. • Supporting the client to do the work. • Evaluation of action taken. • Reviewing the goals ending.	• Goal setting • Action • Planning	Confidence

TREATMENT AND GOAL

1. Classifying the needs and expectations
2. Describe the symptoms (normalize the situation)
3. Prescribing the task (awareness, when to fight)
4. Relabeling of behaviors (put A positive)
5. Engaged in problem solving and negotiation for change.

TYPES OF COUNSELING

- Directive counseling.
- Non-directive counseling or client centered counseling.
- Short term counseling.
- Long term counseling.
- Elective counseling.
- Clinical counseling.
- Psychological counseling.
- Psychotherapeutic counseling.
- Vocational counseling.
- Individual or group counseling.
- Marriage counseling.
- Behavioral counseling.
- Motivational counseling.
- Interpersonal couseling.
- Problem solving counseling.
- Self help group counseling.
- Peer group counseling.

METHODS OF COUNSELING

1. Ventilation
2. Explanation
3. Reassurance
4. Diverssion by physical and mental activities
5. Recreation
6. Improve the problem solving skills
7. Encourage healthy defence mechanism
8. Suggestion
9. Reinforcement
10. Get support from significant other
11. Change of attitude and lifestyle.

Chapter 9

FIELD TRIP AND OBSERVATIONAL VISIT

OUTPATIENT DEPARTMENT MODULE

FUNCTIONS OF OPD

Basic front desk module which assigns each patient with a unique lifetime registration ID to enable easy data retrieval anytime.

Registration contains all mandatory demographic details of the patient.

Registration can be for general patients, for corporate clients as well as staff / scheme enrollees. Updating/editing of data easily done through the screens.

Registration can be for clinical consultation, diagnostics, corporate health check-ups, immunization camps etc & are cross linked with referring doctors, visit details, appointments scheduled, etc.

At glance info of appointments taken, confirmations, rescheduling possible from reception/registration desk.

Consultant's details maintained in a separate database.

Appointment scheduling for clinicians, diagnostics incorporated.

Billing is part of the module so as to enable bill generation & cash management at the reception counter.

Trend analysis possible on various details of the patient as well as consultants, e.g., MIS detailed reporting on patient specifics, clinician's performance, utilization etc.

The Outpatient Department System includes the following modules

1. Central Registration
2. Appointments
3. Reception and Enquiry Help
4. Billing and Cash Management
5. Management Information System (MIS).

MENTAL RETARDATION REHABILITATION

INTRODUCTION

Mental health professionals and members of the community in response to the felt need for the provision of after care and rehabilitative services for the severed and chronically mentally ill and disabled.

GOAL

Objectives of rehabilitation, research and public education in the field of chronic mental illness through very specific and pragmatic programmes aimed at disability reduction/ prevention which are eclectic in their use of a variety of techniques.

REHABILITATION SETTINGS

DAY CARE: This involves basically the use of four modules: Medication management, occupational/vocational rehabilitation, social skills training, and family management. Medication management follows an elaborate procedure of case work by a multi-disciplinary team of psychiatrists, psychiatric social workers and psychologists. Apart from a detailed personal, illness related and family history, two important parameters are assessed at or soon after intake. They are DISABILITY, which also gives an understanding of the abilities of the individual and SOCIAL FUNCTIONING.

Rehabilitation Plan

A comprehensive rehab, plan is drawn up soon after registration. Those clients requiring intensive case management are prioritized for immediate attention. The areas of focus may be symptom alleviation, family support and guidance, employment/ home-making/education, social skills or cognitive functioning.

Vocational Units

There are units for men and women at the day care centre. Chalk and Phenyl are made and sold in the open market and in schools. A few clients are trained in screen printing, while the better functioning are engaged in the out patient department, and in the administrative office for typing and computer work. Cash incentives are awarded based on set criteria. More than preparing them for specific vocations of life, a definite work habit is inculcated in them, which helps them to function in open employment.

Employment Cell

Placing the improved mentally disabled in open employment Ts~ no mean task. The employment cell maintains a register of "employable" clients and makes sincere attempts to place them in open employment.

Social Skills Training

Is offered in individual and group sessions using several indigenous methods. Keeping in mind the needs of the clients and the families, their background etc., the programmes required are prioritised and offered in that sequence. There is greater emphasis on groups dealing with ADL (activities of daily living) and communication and self care. The families are involved in these programmes so that the training can be continued at home also.

Cognitive Assessment

Involves an understanding of the basic cognitive processes such as the level of comprehension, attention, concentration, judgement etc. A battery of simple and computer based tests are used. If definite deficits are identified, the psychologist undertakes to expose these clients to a programme designed at enhancing these functions.

Family Management

A high premium is paid to the involvement of the families in treatment programmes, considering that they are a critical resource in this country.

To offered an extensive educational programme on various aspects of the illness and its management. This is often followed by an open group session during which they are encouraged to talk to each other. Regular reviews always involve the families, who receive inputs and brochures on various issues as crisis management, medication management etc.

Another important element of family support is the **sponsorship of the education of children** of those too disabled to work. Recreation, yoga and leisure activities are conducted on a regular basis. All important festivals are celebrated with involvement of clients and students of social work.

Residential Rehabilitation Centers

For some clients, a short period of admission into a residential rehab facility becomes imperative. This not only removes them from their environment, but introduces them into a non-intrusive, empathetic and supportive one.

The other center for young, disabled men

- Community home

Community Based Rehabilitation (CBR)

It has been identified the world over, that in the face of limited manpower and fiscal resources, the CBR is the most satisfactory strategy to deal with the problems of chronic mentally ill using minimal inputs from mental health professionals.

Other Activities

Regular training programmes to students of social work, psychology, occupational therapy and nursing on principles and practice of psychosocial rehabilitation. Higher levels of such training are being formulated.

A number of booklets have been brought out on subjects as "Crisis management", "Facts for the family", "Medication management" and on residential services.

Links with other national and international agencies working in the field of rehabilitation such as the World Association for Psychosocial Rehabilitation.

CONCLUSION

There is a world wide awakening to the importance of rehabilitation for the mentally disabled. Testimony to this is the consensus statement of the World Health Organization issued in 1996 which defines psychosocial rehabilitation as "a process that facilitates the opportunity for individuals - who are impaired, disabled or handicapped by a mental disorder - To reach their optimal level of independent functioning in the community. It implies both improving individual's competencies and introducing environmental changes in order to create a life of the best quality possible...".

Another milestone is the recognition by both the state and central governments of the "DISABILITY PRODUCED BY MENTAL ILLNESS". This has now been placed on par with other handicaps. It is now upto the mental health professionals, the families of the disabled and the community at large to see that it gets translated into specific programmes and trickles down to those who deserve it at the grass root level.

PSYCHIATRIC REHABILITATION

DEFINITION

Rehabilitation is "an attempt to provide the best possible community role which will enable the patient to achieve the maximum range of activity, interest and of which he is capable".

—Maxwell Jones (1952)

INDICATIONS

1. Chronic schizophrenia.
2. Chronic organic mental disorders.
3. Mental retardation.
4. Alcohol and drug dependence.

APPROACHES

- Psychoeducation.
- Working with families.

- Group therapy.
- Social skill training.

STEPS

A. Reduction of impairment.
B. Remedication of disabilities through skill training.
C. Remediating disabilities through supportive interventions.
D. Remedication of handicaps.

REHABILITATION TEAM

Psychiatrist, clinical psychologist, psychiatric social worker, psychiatric nurse, occupational therapist, counselor and other mental health paraprofessionals.

ROLE OF NURSE

- Assess the individual strengths, motivation, interpersonal skills, self esteem, activities of daily living and drug compliance.
- Planning and implementation focuses on fostering independence by maximizing personal strengths.
- Find ways for the patient to overcome any remaining impaired areas of functioning.
- Interventions involves therapeutic community, recreational therapy, social skills training and training in basic living skills.
- Evaluation takes place at the level of the impact on the patient, family and the effectiveness of the community service system.

DE-ADDICTION

INTRODUCTION

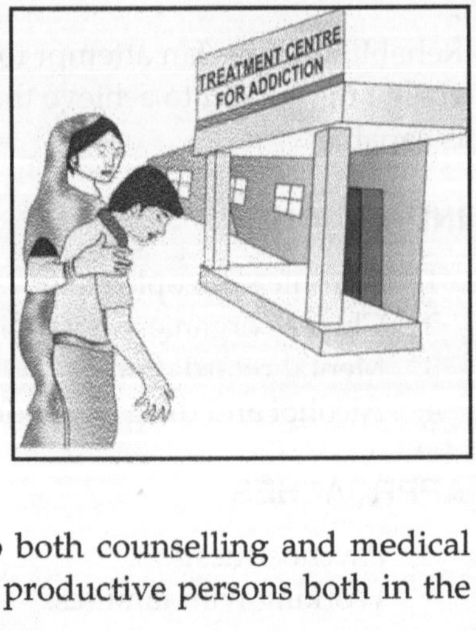

The Aim of this project centre is to eradicate and prevent drug addiction among the people of society. Drug abuse is a psycho-socio-medical problem, which need to be treated in the entirety of the life situations in the addicts. The methodology aims at strengthening the family as a unit and seeks to generate cooperation through motivating addicts to accept detoxification and maintain thereafter a drug free life.

OBJECTIVES

- To cover 200 alcoholics every year to undergo both counselling and medical process and enable them to become better and productive persons both in the family and the society.

- To promote integrated awareness about the ill effects and the havoc behind the problem of alcoholism and substance abuse among the youth in the colleges and the schools.
- To promote happy families with alcoholic free parents through education and treatment in a family setting.
- To undertake researches and study manuals on the problems of alcoholics and their societal status.
- To free people from the habit of drinking and drugs.
- To make them new citizens with fresh memories, thoughts, feelings and experience.

ACTIVITIES

Earlier, people believed that alcoholism was the symptom of some other mental disorder. After extensive research, it has now been established that alcoholism is a disease in itself. A Disease that can be controlled by medical and psychological treatment. Deaddiction centre is dedicated to the treatment and rehabilitation of those addicted to the alcohol and other drugs. It offers a comprehensive in patient treatment program. It includes the involvement of the family of the addict also. Treatment utilizes a multi-disciplinary approach with the help of a psychiatrist, physicians, psychologists, counsellors and social workers. The treatment program includes:

- Detoxification
- Intensive psychological therapy
- Follow-up

The clinical services consist of inpatient and outpatient consultations for alcoholics. It offer comprehensive treatment programme, which includes components of motivation enhancement, relapse prevention, group therapy and family intervention and other psychological interventions. Providing aftercare and more accessible services closer to the community has been one of the major efforts with a focus on developing community responses. It is actively involved in running prevention programmes in rural areas and urban slums, stressing on early identification and brief intervention.

FURTHER READING

1. Ahuja Niraj. *A Short Text Book of Psychiatry*, 3rd ed., Japee Brothers; New Delhi, 1999.
2. Bellack AS Hersen, M, Kazdin AE. *International Handbook of Behaviors Modification and Therapy*. Plenum Press New York, 1982.
3. Bhatia MS. *A Concised Text Book on Psychiatric Nursing*, 1st ed., CBS Publishers New Delhi, 1997.
4. Bimla Kapoor. *Text Book of Psychiatric Nursing*, 1st ed., Kumar Publishing House. New Delhi.
5. Boyd AM. *Psychiatric Nursing Contemporary Practice*. Lippincott-Raven Publishers. New York, 1998.
6. Fink M. *Convulsive Therapy: Theory and Practice*. Raven Press. New York, 1979.
7. Gelder M, Gath D, Mayou R, Cowen P, Oxford University Press: New York, 1996.
8. Heilman KM, Valenstein E. Eds. *Clinical Neuro Psychology*. 2nd ed., Oxford University Press. New York, 1985.
9. Kaplan HI, Sadock BJ, Grebb JA. *Synopsis of Psychiatry*. 8th ed., Williams and Wilkins, 1998.
10. Leff JP, Issacs AD. *Psychiatric Examiniation in Clinical Practice*. 2nd ed., Black Well. Oxford, 1981.
11. Malrika, K. *Psychological Therapy with Children and Adolescents*, NIMHANS, Bangalore.
12. Morrison M. *Foudation of Mental Health Nursing*. Mosby: Philadelphia, 1997.
13. Namboodiri VMD, John CJ, Subulakshmi TP. *Clinical Methods in Psychiatry*. 2nd ed., Churchill Living Stone: New Delhi.
14. Rawlins RP, Williams SR. *Mental Health Psychiatric Nursing –A Holistic Life Cycle Approach*, 3rd ed., CV Mosby: Toronto, 1993.
15. Sadock BJ, Sadock VA. Eds. *Comprehensive Text Book of Psychiatry*. 7th ed., Williams and Wilkins.
16. Schultz MJ, Videbeck LS. *Lippincott's Manual of Psychiatric Nursing Care Plans*, 6th ed., Lippincott Williams and Wilkins Philadelphia, 2002.
17. Slater E, Roth M. *Clinical Psychiatry* (Mayer-Gross). 3rd ed., JPB Publishers. New Delhi, 1986.
18. Stuart WG, Laria TM. *Principles and Practice of Psychiatric Nursing*, 7th ed. Harcourt Private Limited. New Delhi, 2001.

19. Stuart WG, Sundeen JS. *Principles and Practice of Psychiatric Nursing*. 5th ed. C.V Mosby London, 1995.
20. Taylor CM. *Comprehensive Text Book of psychiatry*, 14th ed. C.V Mosby London, 1982.
21. Walsh K. *Neuro Psychology: A Clinical Approach*, 3rd ed. BI Churchill Living Stone. New Delhi, 1994.
22. Wolberg LR. *The Technique of Psychotherapy*. Vol. I and II. Secker and Warburg with Heinemann, London, 1989.

Index